OXFORD MEDICAL PUBLICATIONS
COMMISSION OF THE EUROPEAN COMMUNITIES

Statistical Analysis and Mathematical Modelling of AIDS

Statistical Analysis and Mathematical Modelling of AIDS

Edited by

J.C. Jager and E.J. Ruitenberg

OXFORD   NEW YORK   TOKYO
OXFORD UNIVERSITY PRESS
1988

Oxford University Press, Walton Street, Oxford OX2 6DP

Oxford   New York   Toronto
Delhi   Bombay   Calcutta   Madras   Karachi
Petaling Jaya   Singapore   Hong Kong   Tokyo
Nairobi   Dar es Salaam   Cape Town
Melbourne   Auckland

and associated companies in
Berlin   Ibadan

Oxford is a trade mark of Oxford University Press

Published in the United States
by Oxford University Press, New York

British Library Cataloguing in Publication Data

Statistical analysis and mathematical
modelling of AIDS.
1. Man. AIDS. Epidemiology
I. Jager J. C.   II. Ruitenberg, E. J.
614.5'993
ISBN 0-19-261745-1

Library of Congress Cataloging in Publication Data

Statistical analysis and mathematical modelling of AIDS.
(Oxford medical publications)
The result of a workshop sponsored by the Working Party on AIDS of the European
Communities, held at the National Institute of Public Health and Environmental Hygiene,
Bilthoven, The Netherlands, December 15-17, 1986.
Includes bibliographies and index.
1. AIDS (Disease)——Epidemiology——Statistical
methods——Congresses. 2. AIDS (Disease)——Epidemiology——
Mathematical models——Congresses. 1. Jager, J. C.
II. Ruitenberg, E. J.   III. Commission of the
European Communities. Subgroup Epidemiology.
IV. Series.
RA644.A25S72   1988   614.5'99792'072   88-9913
ISBN 0-19-261745-1

Printed and bound in Great Britain by
Biddles Ltd, Guildford and King's Lynn

Preface

This book is the result of a workshop on the statistical analysis and mathematical modelling of the acquired immunodeficiency syndrome (AIDS) epidemic, which is caused by infections with the human immunodeficiency virus (HIV). The workshop was held at the National Institute of Public Health and Environmental Hygiene, Bilthoven, The Netherlands, 15-17 December 1986. It was organized under the auspices of the Working Party on AIDS of the European Communities (EC). Epidemiology of AIDS (prevention and control) represents one of the major research areas selected for stimulation by the concerted action of the EC in its fight against AIDS. The relevant activities are executed by the Subgroup Epidemiology.

AIDS was first described in the USA in 1981.[1] Using the strict clinical criteria developed by the Centers for Disease Control (CDC), US Public Health Service, over 2500 cases had been diagnosed as of mid-October 1983. More than 1100 of these cases were diagnosed in the first months of 1983 alone. Efforts to locate retrospectively diagnosed cases showed that the syndrome, at least in the epidemic form, was new to the USA, with the earliest cases coming to diagnosis in 1979.[2]

The AIDS outbreak in the USA provoked widespread interest among European clinicians, and soon reports of similar cases began to appear from centres in different parts of Europe. The 'AIDS in Europe, Status Quo 1983' meeting, sponsored jointly by the European Regional Office of the World Health Organization (WHO) and the Danish Society, October 1983, provided the first European opportunity to collect 200 cases of AIDS and to establish guidelines for the collection of further data about AIDS that would be of epidemiological importance. The EC workshop on epidemiology, December 1984, held at the National Institute of Public Health and Environmental Hygiene (Bilthoven) proposed co-ordination and integration of surveillance studies. The WHO Collaborating Centre on AIDS (Paris) was charged with the surveillance of basic epidemiological data. The present workshop on statistical analysis and mathematical modelling of AIDS regards one of the research projects which were initiated by the Subgroup Epidemiology of the EC Working Party on AIDS.

As the doubling time of the numbers of AIDS cases in the USA was as long

---

[1] J.W. Curran, AIDS—two years later. *New Engl. J. Med.* **309**, 609–11, (1983).

[2] M.S. Gottlieb, J.E. Groopman, W.M. Weinstein, J.L. Fahey, R. Detels, The acquired immunodeficiency syndrome. *Am. Intern. Med.* 99, 200–20, (1983).

as nine months, it took the US experts several years fully to realize the steep rise in the curve of reported full-blown AIDS cases. At the EC workshop on immunology in AIDS, Copenhagen, Statens Seruminstitut, October 1984, Dr L'age-Stehr from the German Bundesgesundheitsamt showed with two superposed transparencies the curve for AIDS cases in the USA and the curve in the Federal Republic of Germany, on a semi-logarithmic scale. The inclination angle for both the USA and German curves was roughly equal, the main difference being a time lag of three years. The data published by the WHO Collaborating Centre on AIDS in Paris for the first years of the epidemic in the EC confirmed the predictive potential of the course observed in the USA. Although data are much more scanty for Africa, one is led to believe that similar results hold for Africa, however now with an advance of several years with respect to the USA. In the USA in 1986 the number of reported cases exceeded 25 000 AIDS cases, and the number of persons with the AIDS related complex (ARC), depending on the definition adopted, was between 50 000 and 125 000.

Among homosexual and bisexual men in certain US cities as many as 70 per cent were infected, while for IV drug users precise figures were lacking. In November 1986 the Institute of Medicine and the National Academy of Sciences, independently from any government pressure, regarded their duty to interrupt silence and to warn both the government and public regarding the HIV epidemic. They published jointly a 'shocking' book entitled *Confronting AIDS. Directions for public health, health care, and research* (National Academy Press, Washington D.C. 1986). One expected more than 270 000 cases of AIDS in the USA by the end of 1991. At its meeting of November 1984 the EC Working Party on AIDS through a motion warned that Europe 'was only on the brink of a serious epidemic which will eventually afflict 10 per cent or more of the population. The high population density and morbidity in Europe poses an additional risk for the spread of the disease. Without forceful intervention, supported by clinical and fundamental research at European Community level, the situation will deteriorate and may reach the unmanageable proportions already attained in Central Africa' (Paris, 23 November 1984, unpublished). Initial surveillance studies[1] in Central Africa reported an annual incidence of AIDS of 550 to 1000 cases per million adults. Here the disease was predominantly transmitted by heterosexual activity, exposure to blood transfusion and unsterilized needles, and perinatally from infected mothers to their newborns. These alarming observations from the USA, from Central Africa, and from Europe showed that AIDS represents a serious international infectious disease problem.

An efficient methodology for prediction of future AIDS cases and the

---

[1] T.C. Quinn, J.M. Mann, J.W. Curran, P. Piot, AIDS in Africa: an epidemiologic paradigm. *Science* **234**, 955–63, (1986).

spread of HIV infections, for quantitative evaluations of possible interventions is needed for decisions on public health and the choice of control strategies. Motivated choices of control strategies to minimize the transmission of HIV have to take into account medical, psychosocial, and economic information. Mathematical modelling techniques can help to integrate this information into an efficient methodology for the prediction of future cases, the quantitative evaluation of possible interventions, and associated cost–benefit effects. Detailed discussions and exchange of ideas by epidemiologists, bio-mathematicians, and public health specialists are required for the development of optimal links between data collection—epidemiological surveillance, epidemiological field studies, sociocultural and behavioural studies, information on the natural history of the disease, and its economic impact—and model building, model testing, and model application.

The main purpose of the present workshop is to induce and to stimulate the integration of epidemiological, statistical, and mathematical (model building) research directed to the description, prediction, and simulation of the course of the AIDS epidemic. These proceedings provide only the methodological studies, which were presented at the workshop. Papers on the current situation of the epidemic were dropped because of the temporary character of the fastly changing epidemiological patterns.

The studies in this book and the (rather few) studies on the mathematical approach of AIDS mentioned by the authors, present an overview of the main quantitative techniques available five years after the first recognition of AIDS in the USA. It is hoped that also because of this historical aspect these early studies on the mathematical approach to AIDS may be of interest. Further research to improve use, reliability, and applicability of the mathematical techniques is certainly needed. This research has to be directed to the efficient use of available data, to the integration of data collection (study designs) and model building with the help of statistical techniques (parameter estimation). A wide diversity of models will be needed to cope with the many transmission processes of HIV infections related to risk groups within specified sociocultural and geographic settings. The link of epidemiological models with economic models will deserve special attention.

We should finally like to take this opportunity of thanking R.M. Anderson (London) and K. Dietz (Tübingen) for their advice during the set-up of the workshop and for their critical and detailed comments on the modelling studies. We also acknowledge G. Roumans for typing substantial parts of the manuscript.

Bilthoven   J.C. Jager
1988   A.E. Baert
                                              E.J. Ruitenberg

Contents

Contributors

R.A. Ancelle WHO Collaborating Centre on AIDS, Hôpital Claude Bernard, 10 Avenue Porte d'Aubervilliers, 75019 Paris, France

A.E. Baert Commission of the European Communities, 200 Rue de la Loi, DG XII/F/3 (SDM 2/46), 1049 Brussels, Belgium

Th. de Boo University of Nijmegen, Department of Statistical Consultation (MSA), Toernooiveld 1, 6525 ED Nijmegen, The Netherlands

J.M. Bos National Institute of Public Health and Environmental Hygiene (RIVM), P.O. Box 1, 3720 BA Bilthoven, The Netherlands

J-B. Brunet WHO Collaborating Centre on AIDS, Hôpital Claude Bernard, 10 Avenue Porte d'Aubervilliers, 75019 Paris, France

C. Caroni National Technical University, Athens, Greece

R.A. Coutinho, Municipal Health Service, P.O. Box 20244, 1000 HE Amsterdam, The Netherlands

H. Deicher Zentrum Innere Medizin, Abt. Immunologie, Medizinische Hochschdule Hannover, D-3000 Hannover 61, Federal Republic of Germany

K. Dietz Institute of Medical Biometry, Eberhard-Karls-University, Westbahnhofstrasse 55, D-7400 Tübingen, Federal Republic of Germany

M.G.W. Dijkgraaf Interfacultaire Werkgroep Homostudies, University of Utrecht, Heidelberglaan 1, 3584 CS Utrecht, The Netherlands

D. Dörner Institute of Psychology, University of Bamberg, D-8600 Bamberg, Federal Republic of Germany

A.M. Downs WHO Collaborating Centre on AIDS, Hôpital Claude Bernard, 10 Avenue Porte d'Aubervilliers, 75019 Paris, France

J.A.M. van Druten University of Nijmegen, Department of Statistical Consultation (MSA), Tournooiveld 1, 6525 ED Nijmegen, The Netherlands

J.L.A. Geurts Sociological Institute, University of Nijmegen Tournooiveld 200, 6525 ED Nijmegen, The Netherlands

J.J. Gonzalez Agder College of Engineering, N-4890 Grimstad, Norway

G.J.P. van Griensven Interfacultaire Werkgroep Homostudies, University of Utrecht, Heidelberglaan 1, 3584 CS Utrecht, The Netherlands

S.H. Heisterkamp National Institute of Public Health and Environmental Hygiene (RIVM), P.O. Box 1, 3720 BA Bilthoven, The Netherlands

J.C. Jager National Institute of Public Health and Environmental Hygiene (RIVM), P.O. Box 1, 3720 BA Bilthoven, The Netherlands

A.M. Johnson Academic Department of Genitourinary Medicine, James Pringle House, Middlesex Hospital Medical School, 73–75 Charlotte Street, London WIN 8AA, United Kingdom

D. Kiessling Zentrum Innere Medizin, Abt. Pneumologie, Medizinische Hochschule Hannover, D-3000 Hannover 61, Federal Republic of Germany

E.G. Knox Department of Social Medicine, University of Birmingham, Edgbaston, Birmingham B15 2TJ, United Kingdom

M.G. Koch Skaraborg Läns Landsting, Vårdcentralen (VåC), Box 3009, S-54600 Karlsborg, Sweden

J.L'age-Stehr National Reference Centre of AIDS Epidemiology, Bundes-gesundheitsamt, Robert Koch-Institute, Nordufer 20, D-1000 Berlin 65, Federal Republic of Germany

L.E. Lieb County of Los Angeles, Department of Health Services, 313 North Figueroa Street, Los Angeles, CA 90012, USA

M. Myrtveit SIMSIM, N-5120 Manger, Bergen, Norway

G. Papaevangelou National Centre for AIDS, Athens School of Hygiene, P.O. Box 14085, Athens 11521, Greece

J. Pickering Department of Entomology, University of Georgia, Athens, GA 30602, USA

A.G.M. Reintjes University of Nijmegen, Department of Statistical Consul-tation (MSA), Toernooiveld 1, 6525 ED Nijmegen, The Netherlands

S.C. Richardson National Centre for AIDS, Athens School of Hygiene, P.O. Box 14085, Athens 11521, Greece

E.J. Ruitenberg National Institute of Public Health and Environmental Hygiene (RIVM), P.O. Box 1, 3720 BA Bilthoven, The Netherlands

G.W. Rutherford City and County of San Francisco, Department of Public Health, AIDS Office, 111 Market Street, San Francisco, CA 94103, USA

I. Schedel Zentrum Innere Medizin, Abt. Immunologie Medizinische Hoch-schule Hannover, D-3000 Hannover 61, Federal Republc of Germany

S. Stannat Zentrum Innere Medizin, Abt. Immunologie Medizinische Hoch-schule Hannover, D-3000 Hannover 61, Federal Republic of Germany

H.E. Tillett Public Health Laboratory Service, Communicable Diseases Surveillance Centre, 61 Colindale Avenue, London NW9 5EQ, United Kingdom

L. Vavik Stord Teachers' College, N-5414 Rommetveit, Norway

J. Walker The City of New York, Department of Health, 125 Worth Street, Box 44, New York NY 10013, USA

J.A. Wiley, Survey Research Center and San Francisco Men's Health Study, University of California, Berkeley, CA 94720, USA

Workshop participants

This book is the result of an EC Workshop on Statistical Analysis and Mathematical Modelling of AIDS, held at the National Institute of Public Health and Environmental Hygiene (RIVM), Bilthoven, The Netherlands, 15–17 December, 1986. The following were participants.

R. van den Akker National Institute of Public Health and Environmental Hygiene (RIVM), P.O. Box 1, 3720 BA Bilthoven, The Netherlands

R.A. Ancelle WHO Collaborating Centre on AIDS, Hôpital Claude Bernard, 10 Avenue Porte d'Aubervilliers, 75019 Paris, France

R.M. Anderson Department of Pure and Applied Biology, Imperial College of Science and Technology, University of London, Prince Consort Road, London SW7 2BB, United Kingdom

R. de Andres-Medina Instituto de Salud Carlos III, Unidad de SIDA (CNMVIS), Majadahonda, 28220 Madrid, Spain

A.E. Baert Commission of the European Communities, 200 Rue de la Loi, DG XII/F/3 (SDM 2/46), 1049 Brussels, Belgium

N.T.J. Bailey Division d'Informatique Medicale, Hopital Cantonal Universitaire de Genéve, 24 Rue Michel du Crest, CH-1211 Geneva 4, Switzerland

E.C. Beuvery National Institute of Public Health and Environmental Hygiene (RIVM), P.O. Box 1, 3720 BA Bilthoven, The Netherlands

H. Bijkerk Division of Infectious Diseases, State Supervision of Public Health, Ministry of Welfare, Health and Cultural Affairs, P.O. Box 5406, 2280 HK Rijswijk, The Netherlands

J.L. Boldsen Odense University, Institute of Community Health, Department of Social Medicine, J.B. Winsløws Vej 17, DK-5000, Odense C, Denmark

Th. de Boo University of Nijmegen, Department of Statistical Consultation (MSA), Tournooiveld 1, 6525 ED Nijmegen, The Netherlands

J.M. Bos National Institute of Public Health and Environmental Hygiene (RIVM), P.O. Box 1, 3720 BA Bilthoven, The Netherlands

M. Böttiger Statens Bakteriologiska Laboratorium (SBL), Lundagatan 2, Solna, 10521 Stockholm, Sweden

G. Burchard Bernhard-Nocht-Institut für Schiffs- und Tropenkrankheiten,

Bernhard-Nocht-Strasse 74, 2000 Hamburg 4, Federal Republic of Germany

B.D. Bytchenko Regional Officer for Communicable Diseases (WHO), Scherfigsvej 8, 2100 Copenhagen, Denmark

M.A.E. Conijn-van Spaendonck National Institute of Public Health and Environmental Hygiene (RIVM), P.O. Box 1, 3720 BA Bilthoven. The Netherlands

R.A. Coutinho Municipal Health Service, P.O. Box 20244, 1000 HE Amsterdam, The Netherlands

E. Declerq University of Louvain in Brussels, EPID/3034, Clos Chapelle aux Champs 30, 1200 Brussels, Belgium

E.L. van Dedem Medical Vaccine Affairs, National Institute of Public Health and Environmental Hygiene (RIVM), P.O. Box 1, 3720 BA Bilthoven, The Netherlands

V. Degruttola Harvard University, Department of Biostatistics, 677 Huntington Avenue, Boston, MA 02115, USA

K. Dietz Institut fúr Medizinische Biometrie, Universität Tübingen, Westbahnhofstrasse 55, D-7400 Tübingen, Federal Republic of Germany

M.G.W. Dijkgraaf Interfacultaire Werkgroep Homostudies, University of Utrecht, Heidelberglaan 1, 3584 CS Utrecht, The Netherlands

J.W. Dorpema National Institute of Public Health and Environmental Hygiene (RIVM), P.O. Box 1, 3720 BA Bilthoven, The Netherlands

A.M. Downs WHO Collaborating Centre on AIDS, Hôpital Claude Bernard, 10 Avenue Porte d'Aubervilliers, 75019 Paris, France

J.A.M. van Druten, University of Nijmegen, Department of Statistical Consultation (MSA), Tournooiveld 1, 6525 ED Nijmegen, The Netherlands

J.D.A. van Embden Laboratory for Bacteriology, National Institute for Public Health and Environmental Hygiene (RIVM), P.O. Box 1, 3720 BA Bilthoven, The Netherlands

H.W.B. Engel Laboratory of Parasitology and Mycology, National Institute of Public Health and Environmental Hygiene (RIVM), P.O. Box 1, 3720 BA Bilthoven, The Netherlands

J.T. Garcia Instituto Nacional de Saúde, Av. Padre Cruz, 1699 Lisbon, Portugal

J.J. Gonzalez Agder College of Engineering, N-4890 Grimstad, Norway

G.J.P. van Griensven Interfacultaire Werkgroep Homostudies, Rijksuniversiteit Utrecht, Heidelberglaan 1, 3584 CS Utrecht, The Netherlands

J.D. Griffiths Department of Mathematics, Aberconway Building, University of Wales Institute of Science and Technology, Cardiff CF1 3EU, United Kingdom

A.C. Hekker National Institute of Public Health and Environmental Hygiene (RIVM), P.O. Box 1, 3720 BA Bilthoven, The Netherlands

S.H. Heisterkamp Centre for Mathematical Methods, National Institute of Public Health and Environmental Hygiene (RIVM), P.O. Box 1, 3720 BA Bilthoven, The Netherlands

A. van Hemeldonck Institute of Hygiene and Epidemiology, 14 Rue Juliette Wytsman, 1050 Brussels, Belgium

H. Houweling Department of Epidemiology, National Institute of Public Health and Environmental Hygiene (RIVM), P.O. Box 1, 3720 BA Bilthoven, The Netherlands

S.T. Howard Taylor Nelson Group, 44–46 Upper High Street, Epsom, Surrey KT17 4QS, United Kingdom

G. Ippolito Osservatoro Epidemiologico Regione Lazio, Via Giosne Carducci 4, 00187 Rome, Italy

J.C. Jager Centre of Mathematical Methods, National Institute of Public Health and Environmental Hygiene (RIVM), P.O. Box 1, 3720 BA Bilthoven, The Netherlands

A. Johnson Academic Department of Genitourinary Medicine, James Pringle House, Middlesex Hospital Medical School, 73–75 Charlotte Street, London WIN 8AA, United Kingdom

J. Th. L. Jong Centre for Mathematical Methods, National Institute of Public Health and Environmental Hygiene (RIVM), P.O. Box 1, 3720 BA Bilthoven, The Netherlands

E.G. Knox Department of Social Medicine, University of Birmingham, Edgbaston, Birmingham B15 2TJ, United Kingdom

M.A. Koch Bundesgesundheitsamt, Robert-Koch-Institut, Nordufer 20, D-1000 Berlin 65, Federal Republic of Germany.

M.G. Koch Skaraborgs Läns Landsting, Vårdcentralen (VåC), Box 3009, S-54600 Karlsborg, Sweden

M.J.W. van de Laar Nederlands Instituut voor Praeventieve Gezondheidszorg TNO, P.O. Box 124, 2300 AC Leiden, The Netherlands

S.W. Lagakos Harvard University, Department of Biostatistics, 677 Huntington, Avenue, Boston, MA 02115, USA

J.L'age-Stehr Bundesgesundheitsamt, Robert Koch-Institut, Nordufer 20, D-1000 Berlin 65, Federal Republic of Germany

M.F. Lechat University of Louvain in Brussels, EPID/3034, Clos Chapelle aux Champs, 1200 Brussels, Belgium

A. van Loon Laboratory of Virology, Radboutziekenhuis, Geert Grooteplein, 6525 EZ Nijmegen, The Netherlands

M.B. McEvoy PHLS Communicable Diseases Surveillance Centre, 61 Colindale Avenue, London NW9 5EQ, United Kingdom

M. Myrtveit SIMSIM, N-5120 Manger, Bergen, Norway

A.D.M.E. Osterhaus Viral Vaccine Control, National Institute of Public Health and Environmental Hygiene (RIVM), P.O. Box 1, 3720 BA Bilthoven, The Netherlands

J. Pickering Department of Entomoloyg, University of Georgia, Athens, GA 30602, USA

A.D. Plantinga National Institute of Public Health and Environmental Hygiene (RIVM), P.O. Box 1, 3720 BA Bilthoven, The Netherlands

S.C. Richardson Athens School of Hygiene, Department of Epidemiology and Medical Statistics, National Centre for AIDS, P.O. Box 14085, Athens 11521, Greece

E.J. Ruitenberg National Institute of Public Health and Environmental Hygiene (RIVM), P.O. Box 1, 3720 BA Bilthoven, The Netherlands

H. Rümke National Institute of Public Health and Environmental Hygiene (RIVM), P.O. Box 1, 3720 BA Bilthoven, The Netherlands

H. Scarabis Institut für Soziologie, Babelsbergerstrasse 14/16, 1000 Berlin 31, Federal Republic of Germany

W. Schappacher Institute of Mathematics, University of Graz, Elisabeth Strasse 16, A-8010 Graz, Austria

I. Schedel Zentrum Innere Medizin, Abt. Immunologie, Medizinische Hochschule Hannover, D-3000 Hannover 61, Federal Republic of Germany

F. Schneider Department of Bacteriology, Laboratoire National de Santé 42, Rue du Laboratoire, L-1011 Luxembourg-City, Luxembourg

F. Sogaard Institute of Social Medicine, University of Aarhus, 800 Aarhus C, Denmark

S. Stannat Zentrum Innere Medizin, Abt. Immunologie, Medizinische Hochschule Hannover, D-3000 Hannover 61, Federal Republic of Germany

G. van Steenis National Institute of Public Health and Environmental Hygiene (RIVM), P.O. Box 1, 3720 BA Bilthoven, The Netherlands

L.A.M. Stolte Praeventiefonds, Frankenstraat 3, 2582 SC Den Haag, The Netherlands

H.E. Tillett Public Health Laboratory Service, Communicable Diseases Surveillance Centre, 61 Colindale Avenue, London NW9 5EQ, United Kingdom

F. Uytdehaag Bacterial Vaccines, National Institute of Public Health and Environmental Hygiene (RIVM), P.O. Box 1, 3720 BA Bilthoven, The Netherlands

A-J. Valleron Unité de Recherches Biomathématiques et Biostatistiques (URBB), INSERM-U263, Université Paris 7, 75251 Paris, France

L. Vavik Stord Teachers' College, N-5414 Rommetveit, Norway

H. Vorkauf Federal Office of Public Health, Bollwerk 27, CH 3001 Bern, Switzerland

E.M.M. Vroome Interfacultaire Werkgroep Homostudies, University of Utrecht, Heidelberglaan 1, 3584 CS Utrecht, The Netherlands

D. van Waarde Coordinatiecentrum Nederlands Medisch Wetenschappelijk Onderzoek in EG-verband, Koningin Sophiestraat 124, 2595 TM 's-Gravenhage, The Netherlands

H.P.A. van de Water Nederlands Instituut voor Praeventieve Gezondheidszorg TNO, Postbus 124, 2300 AC Leiden, The Netherlands

Frh. Uli V. Welck ACS, Samerhofstrasse 15, D-8000 München 60, Federal Republic of Germany

J. Weyer Mathematisches Institut der Universität Köln, Weyertal 86–90, D-5000 Köln 41, Federal Republic of Germany

K. Wheeler Department of Mathematics, Aberconway Building, University of Wales Institute of Science and Technology, Cardiff CF1 3EU, United Kingdom

J.K. van Wijngaarden AIDS Policy Coordination, Polderweg 92, 1093 KP Amsterdam, The Netherlands

1

The statistical estimation, from routine surveillance data, of past, present, and future trends in AIDS incidence in Europe

A.M. Downs, R.A. Ancelle, J.C. Jager, S.H. Heisterkamp,
J.A.M. van Druten, E.J. Ruitenberg, and J.B. Brunet

1. Introduction

Attempts to predict the future course of an epidemic quantitatively can be based either on a mechanistic mathematical model of the natural history of the disease or on a purely empirical statistical model. These alternative approaches play somewhat different, although complementary, roles and the choice of one or the other type of model is dependent, among other things, on the precise objective in mind. A mathematical model which takes into account the underlying characteristics of the transmission and other properties of the disease is indispensable for the consideration of probable long-term outcomes, including the quantitative assessment of the likely effects of possible intervention strategies. Empirical approaches, in which predictions of future incidence are made by extrapolation from a curve chosen by its ability to fit the pattern of previous observations, are highly dependent for their success on the extent to which currently observed trends continue to operate in the future and are thus most appropriate in connection with relatively short-term predictions. Despite the uncertainties inherent in the extrapolation of past trends into the future, such an approach may represent the only reasonable alternative when an incomplete understanding of the natural history of the disease precludes the setting up of a sufficiently reliable mechanistic model.

Despite the rapid progress made in basic virological research into HIV since its discovery in 1983 as the underlying causative agent of AIDS, many aspects of the transmission and other dynamics of HIV infection in given populations remain poorly understood and unreliably quantified. Estimates of such basic epidemiological parameters as the incubation-time distribution and the proportion of HIV-infected persons who will eventually develop full-blown AIDS are continually being revised upwards as the epidemic progresses and more data, based on longer periods of observation, become

1

available. Other factors, such as the length of the infectious period or the length of time the virus remains within the host, are even less well understood. Thus, although several models based on current knowledge and assumptions concerning the characteristics of HIV infection and disease progression are currently being developed (van Druten, de Boo, Jager, Heisterkamp, Coutinho, and Ruitenberg 1986; Knox 1986; Kiessling, Stannat, Schedel, and Deicher 1986; Pickering, Wiley, Padian, Lieb, Echenberg, and Walker 1986; Anderson, Medley, May, and Johnson 1986) (see also other contributions to these *Proceedings*) these should be regarded, for the time being, as tools for purposes such as exploring alternative possible scenarios and assessing which parameters are likely to be most critical. As stressed by Anderson *et al.* (1986), the use of such models to generate reliable predictions of future trends in AIDS incidence seems premature.

In addition to providing quantitative descriptions of the evolution and current trends of the epidemic, the statistical analysis of AIDS surveillance data would thus appear to remain the most reasonable approach, at the present time, to the provision of short-term predictions. Furthermore, estimates of initial epidemic growth rates and their subsequent evolution in particular geographical and/or behavioural subgroups can be of use in the construction and validation of mechanistic models.

2. The use of surveillance data

Since its creation in 1984, the WHO Collaborating Centre in Paris has been receiving regular reports from a steadily increasing number of European countries. The Centers for Disease Control (CDC) case definition of AIDS is used and information is supplied to the Paris Centre on standardized forms by one nationally recognized source per country. At regular three-monthly intervals each participating country reports total cumulated numbers of AIDS cases by risk group, by geographic origin and place of residence, and independently by half-year period of diagnosis from 1981 onwards. The Centre produces a quarterly report summarizing and commenting upon the current situation (WHO Collaborating Centre on AIDS 1987).

At the outset of the surveillance scheme, date (half-year) of diagnosis was selected as the time variable for the enumeration of cases on the grounds that it was the least ambiguous and the least subject to variance among several possible choices (e.g. date of first symptoms, date of first medical consultation) and this remains the most natural choice as independent variable in a regression analysis. However, as with any disease-reporting system, there are frequently significant delays between the diagnosis and the reporting of cases so that, at any given time, an unknown number of cases is already diagnosed but not yet reported. This problem is further exacerbated by a dual reporting system, with cases being first reported to national surveillance centres and subsequently to the Paris Centre. With date of diagnosis as independent variable, straightforward use of all the most recently reported data would thus result in an underestimation of the epidemic growth rate. Three possible procedures were considered: the use of reporting date rather than date of diagnosis as independent variable, the exclusion of the most recently diagnosed cases, and the use of adjusted data. There is evidence that, at least for some countries, case reports are sometimes clustered, so that reported incidence is not necessarily a good (time-lagged) reflection of diagnosed incidence. The waste of potentially very valuable information if recently diagnosed cases are excluded is also highly undesirable. We therefore opt to work with reported numbers of cases by half-year of diagnosis, adjusted to allow for estimated reporting delays. This approach has also been adopted by Morgan and Curran (1986) in their treatment of surveillance data from the USA, although our method of adjustment differs from theirs in at least one important respect (see Section 5).

McEvoy and Tillett (1985), in an early attempt at statistical fitting of surveillance data, used an exponential model which appeared to describe well the initial phase of the epidemic in the UK, as was also the case in the USA and elsewhere. It is now fairly clear, however, particularly from experience in the USA (Morgan and Curran 1986; CDC 1986), where the epidemic is more advanced than in Europe, that the subsequent growth is less than exponential, with doubling times observed to be gradually increasing. Other models which have been used include polynomial fitting after Box–Cox transformation (Curran, Morgan, Hardy, Jaffe, Darrow, and Dowdle 1985; Morgan and Curran 1986) and simple quadratic fitting (Artalejo, Albero, Alvarez, Laguarta, and Cabellero 1986). While these or other functional forms may be more successful in fitting the data over the full period of observation to date, they do not necessarily provide a better basis for the assessment of future trends. In particular, as has been pointed out by Gonzalez and Koch (1986), the currently observed incidence rates can be expected to be affected by a negative transient arising from the combination of the (unknown) rate of HIV infection with a broadly distributed incubation period. Extrapolations made from functions chosen to follow too closely the full epidemic curve observed to date could therefore significantly underestimate future numbers of AIDS cases.

Rather than reject the simple exponential model, we therefore chose to examine its fit to the data not only over the complete time period of the epidemic to date but also over successive (overlapping) shorter time periods or 'windows'. This approach has the advantage of yielding directly an estimate of the overall doubling time associated with each time window, thus providing a simple quantitative means of monitoring and comparing the evolution of the epidemic in different countries or groups of countries and for selected risk groups. Short-term predictions can be obtained by extrapolation of the curves fitted to data from the most recent period, i.e. based on an estimated current doubling time.

The methods described here have been applied to data reported to the Paris Centre at the nominal reporting date of 30 June 1986. Some of the final results, which have been presented more fully elsewhere (Downs, Ancelle, Jager, and Brunet 1987), are reproduced here for illustration, together with additional details concerning the preliminary analyses which were made.

3. Methods

3.1. Estimation of reporting delays and adjustment of data

Since cases are reported by half-year period of diagnosis, the half-year was chosen as the basic unit of time and, accordingly, only alternate quarterly reports were used in the analysis.

For any country or group of countries, let n_{ij} be the number of AIDS cases diagnosed in the jth half-year period ($j = 1, 2, \ldots, t$) and *first* reported at reporting time i ($i = s, s+1, \ldots, t$), where t denotes the current time in half-years measured from the start of the epidemic (or from the beginning of 1981, if later) and s denotes the time of the first surveillance report. At any time q ($\geq j$) the total reported incidence N_{qj} of cases diagnosed in the jth period is thus given by

$$N_{qj} = \sum_{i=s}^{q} n_{ij} = \sum_{k=0}^{q-s} n_{q-k, j},$$

where k represents the delay between diagnosis and reporting. Suppose further that the true (unknown) number of cases diagnosed in the jth period is N_j and put

$$r_{kj} = \frac{n_{j+k, j}}{N_{j+k, j}}.$$

The proportion of cases diagnosed in period j which are reported with delay k is then given by

$$p_{kj} = \frac{n_{j+k, j}}{N_j} = \frac{r_{kj} N_{j+k, j}}{N_j} = r_{kj} \prod_{l=k+1}^{\infty} (1 - r_{lj}).$$

where r_{lj} ($j = 1, \ldots, t$) is known for max $\{0, s - j\} \leq l \leq t - j$. If we now assume that the pattern of reporting remains constant with time, we can replace r_{kj} and p_{kj} by r_k and p_k respectively. Assuming also a maximum reporting delay k_{max}, we thus obtain

$$p_k \approx r_k \prod_{l=k+1}^{k_{max}} (1 - r_l) \qquad k = 0, \ldots, k_{max} - 1$$

with $r_0 = 1$ and $p_{kmax} = r_{kmax}$. For any chosen value of k_{max} (in practice, $k_{max} \le t - 1$), estimates of r_k ($1 \le k \le k_{max}$) can be obtained from the data and used to derive estimates $\hat{p}_k$ for the proportion of cases expected to be reported with delay k. The value of r_k was estimated according to

$$r_k = \left(\sum_{l=l_0}^{t-k} n_{l+k, l} \right) \Big/ \sum_{l=l_0}^{t-k} N_{l+k, l},$$

where $l_0 = \max(1, s + 1 - k)$. The latest reported incidence data N_{tj} for recent diagnostic periods can then be adjusted using

$$\hat{N}_j = \frac{N_{tj}}{\displaystyle\sum_{k=0}^{t-j} \hat{p}_k} \qquad t - k_{max} \le j \le t.$$

In applications (Downs *et al.* 1987) we took $k_{max} = 4$ and estimated r_k ($k \le 4$) by pooling data from all diagnostic periods for which the requisite time delay had elapsed, except when a clear disturbance in reporting pattern was evident (owing, for example, to a large-scale reclassification of previously reported cases) in which case only data reported subsequent to this disturbance were used. The procedure was applied to all countries with at least 50 reported cases. To allow their subsequent inclusion in an overall European Community (EC) model, data from those EC countries with less than 50 cases were either adjusted on the basis of average EC delay times or, in the absence of any evidence of reporting delays, left unadjusted.

3.2. Analysis of trends

The extent to which a simple exponential model could be fitted to the adjusted data over the complete time period of the epidemic to date was first examined using the following alternative models:

model 1 ('linear') $\qquad y_j = \ln N_j = \beta_0 + \beta_1 j + \epsilon_j$

and

model 2 ('quadratic') $\quad y_j = \ln N_j = \beta_0 + \beta_1 j + \beta_2 j^2 + \epsilon_j,$

where $N_j (j = 1, \ldots, t)$ is the adjusted number of cases diagnosed in the jth half-year period. In any data set which included a zero value, N_j was systematically replaced by $(N_j + 0.5)$. The adjusted coefficient of determination $\bar{R}^2$ for each model was computed according to the formula

$$\bar{R}^2 = 1 - \frac{n - 1}{n - m - 1} (1 - R^2),$$

where n is the number of observations, m is the number of degrees of freedom for regression and R^2 is the usual coefficient of determination. The use of $\bar{R}^2$ rather than R^2 is preferable when comparing the fits for different countries, as the value of n is not the same in each case (Draper and Smith 1981). Tests of the null hypothesis H_0 ($\beta_2 = 0$) were also carried out. For the linear model, the distribution of the unexplained variation was examined by plotting the residuals as a function of the independent time variable j.

Further regression analyses were then performed using the linear model only over a series of successive and overlapping time windows, each of width n half-year periods (i.e. for $j = j_1, \ldots, j_1 + n - 1$, with $j_1 = 1, \ldots, t - n + 1$) with $n = 6$ in most cases. The doubling time (time for the number of cases to double) in months was estimated for each window as $6 \ln 2 / \hat{\beta}_1$, where $\hat{\beta}_1$ is the least-squares estimate of β_1.

Predictions of the number of cases $\hat{N}_{t+l} = \exp(\hat{y}_{t+l})$, $l = 1, 2, \ldots$ to be expected in future half-yearly periods were made by extrapolation of the regression line fitted over the most recent time window ($j = t - n + 1, \ldots, t$). Corresponding confidence limits for individual half-year predictions were computed from the estimated standard error of $\hat{y}_{t+l}$:

$$s(\hat{y}_{t+l}) = \left\{ 1 + \frac{1}{n} + \frac{(t + l - \bar{j})^2}{\displaystyle\sum_{j=t-h+1}^{t} (j - \bar{j})^2} \right\}^{1/2} s,$$

where s^2 is the mean square deviation from regression and $\bar{j} = \dfrac{1}{n} \displaystyle\sum_{j=t-n+1}^{t} j$

(see, for example, Draper and Smith 1981).

4. Results

Full results of the analysis applied to the data reported to Paris by 30 June 1986, with predictions to mid-1988, are presented and discussed elsewhere (Downs *et al.* 1987), and an update to 31 December 1986 will shortly be available. However, selected results are reproduced below for illustration, together with additional results from the preliminary analyses.

4.1. Reporting delays and data adjustment

Examination of successive 3-monthly reports (up to 30 June 1986) revealed that, for most countries, cases continued to be reported, in quite significant numbers, for up to at least two years following diagnosis (Fig. 1.1(a)). Within this period, the reporting pattern appeared to show considerable variation between countries. It was therefore decided to make separate estimations of the reporting delay probabilities p_k for each country, as described above (with $k_{\max} = 4$). The results are presented in Table 1.1.

Typical effects of applying the adjustment procedure are shown in Fig. 1.1b. To assess the effectiveness of the procedure, data reported at 31 December 1985 were similarly processed and the resulting adjusted data were compared with those reported at the end of June 1986. Overall, the suggested

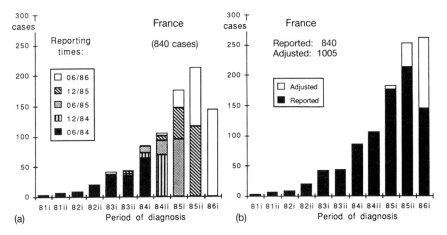

Fig. 1.1. AIDS cases in France (January 1981–June 1986) illustrating a typical reporting pattern and the effect of data adjustment: (a) total cases reported at 30 June 1984 and additional cases reported at 6-monthly intervals to 30 June 1986; (b) as reported at 30 June 1986 and after adjustment.

Table 1.1. Estimated cumulated reporting-delay probabilities based on data reported up to 30 June 1986.

	Reporting delay k in units of 6 months				Cases reported at 30.6.1986 (diagnosed $\geq$ 1981)
	0	1	2	4†	
Belgium	0.42	0.74	0.92	1.00	168
Denmark	0.88	1.00			92
France	0.55	0.84	0.96	1.00	840
FRG	0.77	0.97	1.00		537
Italy	0.46	0.83	0.90	1.00	300
Netherlands	0.72	0.89	0.95	1.00	146
Spain	0.31	0.76	0.90	1.00	177
Sweden	1.00				57
Switzerland	0.71	0.93	1.00		136
UK‡	0.31	0.67	0.90	1.00	344

†Maximum delay of 2 years assumed.
‡Based on reports from June 1985 onwards only.

adjustment seemed to be reasonably satisfactory. For the EC as a whole, 389 cases diagnosed prior to 1 January 1986 were reported for the first time in March or June 1986, compared with the 349 expected. However, France and Spain both reported significantly more back cases than expected, while Belgium and the UK reported considerably less.

Table 1.2.   Adjusted coefficients of determination $\bar{R}^2$ in regression analyses of adjusted data and outcomes of tests of linearity ($H_0:\beta_2 = 0$) from data as reported up to 30 June 1986.

		Onset (or Jan 81)–June 86			July 83–June 86
	n†	$\bar{R}^2$ (linear)	$\bar{R}^2$ (quadratic)	Test outcome	$\bar{R}^2$ (linear)
Belgium	11	0.84	0.91	‡	0.52
Denmark	11	0.95	0.95	NS	0.80
France	11	0.96	0.99	§	0.93
FRG	9	0.94	0.97	‡	0.93
Italy	9	0.93	0.93	NS	0.96
Netherlands	9	0.92	0.93	NS	0.80
Spain	10	0.96	0.96	NS	0.97
Sweden	7	0.74	0.67	NS	0.79
Switzerland	11	0.86	0.84	NS	0.91
UK	11	0.92	0.95	NS	0.89
EC‖	11	0.98	0.99	¶	0.98

NS, not significant.
†Number of time periods available for analysis.
‡$0.01 \leqslant P \leqslant 0.05$.
§$P < 0.001$.
¶$0.001 \leqslant P \leqslant 0.01$.
‖European Community global model (Belgium excluded).

4.2. The regression analyses

Results of the preliminary analyses, using both the linear and quadratic models over the complete time period, are presented in Table 1.2 and Fig. 1.2. Although the use of the quadratic model generally resulted in an improved fit, as measured by the value of $\bar{R}^2$, the difference in fit was, rather surprisingly, found to be significant in only four of the 11 populations investigated. In terms of the 'linear' model, although reasonably good overall fits were obtained for most countries (Table 1.2, Fig. 1.2(a)), visual examination of the residual plots (Fig. 1.2(b)) revealed in most cases a more or less parabolic-like trend, suggestive of a less than exponential rate of increase in the number of cases (i.e. a downward curvature when plotted on a semilogarithmic scale).

This tendency was confirmed by the results obtained from successive time windows (Table 1.3). For the EC as a whole, the estimated doubling time lengthened from 6.5 months to 9.4 months over a period of 2.5 years. Similar evolutions were found in most individual countries investigated, with the notable exceptions of Italy, Spain, and Switzerland. Values of $\bar{R}^2$ for regression over the final time window are included in Table 1.2. The Belgian data

Table 1.3 Epidemic doubling times as estimated from regression analyses over the full period to 30 June 1986 and over successive 3-year time windows.

	Onset (or Jan 81)– June 86	Time windows					
		Jan 81– Dec 83	July 81– June 84	Jan 82– Dec 84	July 82– June 85	Jan 83– Dec 85	July 83– June 86
Belgium	14.9 (11.4, 21.8)	9.6§	9.2§	12.6§	14.6¶	24.2§	(—)¶
Denmark	12.2 (10.5, 14.5)	10.0	8.9	11.7§	12.1¶	14.6§	17.7§
France	8.5 (7.4, 10.1)	6.5	7.3	8.4	9.8	10.6	11.2
FRG	7.9 (6.5, 10.0)	—	—	6.8	8.3	8.4	9.3
Italy	5.3 (4.3, 6.7)	—	—	6.9§	4.6	4.6	4.3
Netherlands	8.7 (7.0, 11.5)	—	—	7.4§	8.5§	10.6¶	10.1§
Spain	7.1 (6.1, 8.5)	—	7.7§	7.1§	6.6	7.1	6.3
Sweden	11.0 (6.8, 27.7)	—	—	—	—	9.9¶	8.9¶
Switzerland	10.0 (8.2, 12.6)	(—)¶	(—)¶	8.9§	10.6	10.0	9.6
UK	10.3 (8.6, 13.0)	7.8§	7.7§	10.2	10.3	14.3	15.0§
EC‖	8.0 (7.3, 8.8)	6.5	7.0	8.4	8.7	9.3	9.4

Estimates of doubling time (95 per cent confidence limits)† (months)

(—)No estimate given in three cases for which $\bar{R}^2 < 0.70$.
† 95% confidence limits in parentheses; see Table 1.2 for values of $\bar{R}^2$.
§ $0.80 \leqslant \bar{R}^2 < 0.90$.
¶ $\bar{R}^2 < 0.80$
‖ European Community global model (Belgium excluded).
In all cases other than those indicated $\bar{R}^2 \geqslant 0.90$.

were not satisfactorily fitted by the exponential model, particularly over the later time windows. This can be explained by the fact that a very high proportion of the early cases diagnosed were among non-residents (mostly of African origin), and this proportion has recently fallen significantly, thus distorting the epidemic curve (see Downs *et al.* 1987). In future, data relating to residents only will be made available for analysis, and it is expected that these will show a trend similar to those of the other countries of Western Europe.

Examples of short-term predictions for individual countries and for the EC as a whole are shown, with 95 per cent confidence limits, in Table 1.4. Cumulated projections to mid-1988 are given without confidence limits: difficulties in their computation arise from the use of the logarithmic transformation in the regression analysis. The overall EC predictions were made using pooled data from its constituent countries (Belgium excepted) in the regression analysis and thus do not represent the sum of the predictions for the individual countries.

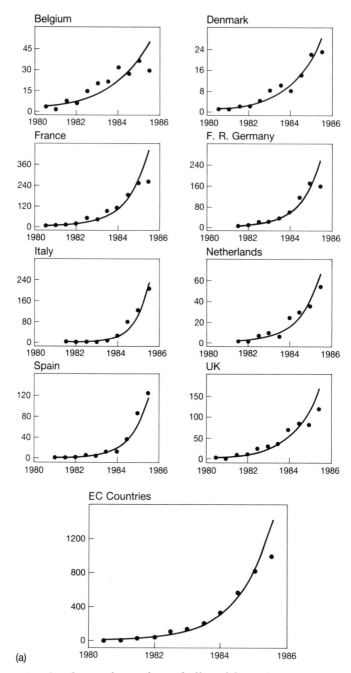

(a)

Fig. 1.2. Results of regression analyses of adjusted data using the 'linear' model (see text) over the complete time period for EC countries with more than 50 reported cases

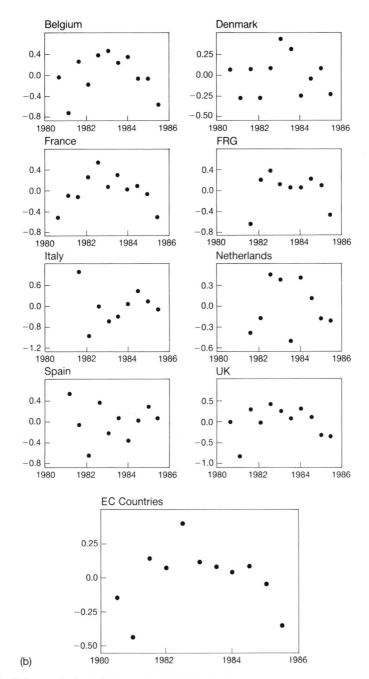

(b)

and the EC as a whole (Belgium excluded): (a) fitted curves and adjusted data points; (b) residual plots.

Table 1.4. AIDS predictions to mid-1988 based on currently estimated doubling times (in parentheses); cases diagnosed prior to 30 June 1986 are also shown.

Country†	Cases diagnosed up to 30.6.86		Cases projected to be diagnosed in half-year periods‡				Cumulated total cases projected diagnosed by 30.6.88
	Rep§	Adj.¶	1986(ii)	1987(i)	1987(ii)	1988(i)	
Denmark (17.7)	93	96	29 (13, 66)	37 (15, 92)	47 (17, 129)	59 (19, 183)	266
France (11.2)	859	1024	471 (228, 974)	683 (304, 1535)	990 (401, 2443)	1434 (525, 3918)	4609
FRG (9.3)	538	580	339 (143, 806)	532 (202, 1397)	834 (284, 2450)	1307 (394, 4335)	3596
Italy (4.3)	300	456	799 (215, 2974)	2094 (483, 9069)	5485 (1068, 28169)	14367 (2328, 88647)	23240
Netherlands (10.1)	146	166	86 (20, 365)	130 (26, 651)	197 (33, 1185)	297 (40, 2190)	874
Spain (6.3)	177	289	265 (118, 595)	512 (208, 1262)	989 (361, 2708)	1910 (623, 5858)	3963
Sweden (8.9)	57	57	34 (7, 177)	54 (9, 341)	87 (11, 672)	138 (14, 1347)	371
Switzerland (9.6)	138	153	81 (32, 205)	124 (44, 352)	191 (60, 612)	295 (81, 1074)	845
UK (15.0)	389	511	165 (84, 326)	218 (102, 465)	288 (123, 671)	380 (148, 974)	1560
EC‖ (9.4)	2736	3184	1774 (1108, 2841)	2756 (1630, 4660)	4282 (2383, 7696)	6653 (3466, 12767)	18690

†Estimated doubling times (in months) in parentheses.
‡Approximate 95 per cent confidence limits in parentheses.
§Reported at 30 June 1986.
¶Adjusted for estimated reporting delays.
‖European Community global model (Belgium excluded).

5. Discussion

An approach to the statistical analysis of AIDS surveillance data with the principal aim of assessing and monitoring trends within particular geographical and/or behavioural subgroups has been described. To best achieve this objective, we have chosen to use all available data including the most recently diagnosed cases, for which reporting is incomplete. This requires that the data be adjusted to allow for delays in reporting.

The adjustment procedure adopted represents an improvement over that used by Morgan and Curran (1986) in that it uses, as the denominator for computing the reporting probabilities p_k, estimates of the true numbers N_j of cases diagnosed in the periods involved, rather than the currently reported numbers N_{tj}. Although not based on an explicitly formulated model, the estimates derived for p_k and N_j can in fact be shown to be numerically identical with the maximum-likelihood estimates for these parameters under the assumption of a Poisson process, given that the same constraint of a maximum reporting delay k_{max} is imposed (Heisterkamp, Jager, Downs, van Druten, and de Boo 1988). Furthermore, comparisons of the numbers of back cases reported from the EC countries between 31 December 1985 and 30 June 1986 with the numbers of such cases expected on the basis of our estimations suggest that the procedure is reasonably satisfactory in practice. Since the estimation of the reporting-delay parameters is based on the assumption that, within a given country, the reporting pattern is relatively stable, the extent to which expected back cases are subsequently reported is partly a reflection of the extent to which reporting practices in the country are changing.

The analysis of reporting delays (Table 1.1) revealed considerable between-country variation, probably reflecting a combination of the differing national structures and traditions of disease reporting in general and differences in attitudes to the reporting of AIDS in particular. It should also be noted that the estimated proportions apply only to those cases which are eventually reported and that no allowance has been made for under-reporting as opposed to delayed reporting of cases. The extent of this problem, which must also vary considerably between countries, is difficult to assess. Although it is generally believed that the reporting of AIDS is better than that of most diseases, it is possible that decreasing rarity and/or other factors may change this situation in the future.

The finding that in most countries doubling times are gradually increasing is in accordance with a similar trend observed in the USA, where doubling times of the number of cases reported to the CDC have increased from around 5 months in January 1982 to around 13 months in December 1986 (CDC 1986). Estimates of current doubling times in Europe (Table 1.3) show considerable variation between countries. This is partly a reflection of the differing commencement times of the epidemic, but other factors, including reporting variability within as well as between countries, and differences in lifestyles, must also play a role. As more data become available, the present approach offers a simple tool for exploring the possibility that the epidemic may be spreading at fundamentally different rates in different risk groups. As reported by Downs *et al.* (1987), preliminary analyses of Italian and French data for the two main risk groups (homosexual/bisexual men and intravenous (IV) drug users) seem to give some support to the idea that the epidemic may spread more rapidly among drug users than among homosexuals. This could explain, at least in part, the short doubling times obtained for Italy and Spain, where IV drug users currently account for roughly 50 per cent of all AIDS cases.

It is suggested that short-term predictions can be made by extrapolation under the exponential model with the estimated current doubling time. However, in view of the evidence that doubling times are continuing to increase, predictions obtained in this way should tend to represent overestimates rather than underestimates, a tendency which should increase as the time interval over which the predictions are made increases. It is our opinion that, at the present time, forecasts cannot reasonably be made for more than 2, or at most 3, years ahead.

Discussion of longer-term aspects, including predictions of the future course which the epidemic could be expected to take in the absence of any effective countermeasures and assessments of the probable effects of specific preventive measures designed to reduce the risk of transmission and/or of intervention strategies such as vaccination (if and when a vaccine becomes available), will require the use of mechanistic models. In the classical approach to the modelling of infectious diseases, a key parameter is the effective contact rate (average number of secondary infected persons generated when one primary infectious individual is introduced into a population of susceptibles). As has been indicated by van Druten *et al.* (1986), estimates of epidemic growth rates in well-defined populations can be used to assess this parameter, which is clearly extremely difficult to measure directly. The ongoing provision of such estimates from surveillance data will thus be of importance for the setting up and validation of future models.

References

Anderson, R.M., Medley, G.F., May, R.M., and Johnson, A.M. (1986). A preliminary study of the transmission dynamics of the human immunodeficiency virus (HIV), the causative agent of AIDS. *IMA Journal of Mathematics Applied in Medicine and Biology* **3**, 229–63.

Artalejo, F.R., Albero, M.J.M., Alvarez, F.V., Laguarta, A.B. and Cabellero, J.G. (1986). Predicting AIDS cases. *Lancet* **i**, 378.

CDC (1986). Update: acquired immunodeficiency syndrome—United States. *MMWR* **35**, 757–66.

Curran, J.W., Morgan, W.M., Hardy, A.M., Jaffe, H.M., Darrow, W.W., and Dowdle, W.R. (1985). The epidemiology of AIDS: current status and future prospects. *Science* **229**, 1352–7.

Downs, A.M., Ancelle, R.A., Jager, J.C., and Brunet, J.B. (1987). AIDS in Europe: current trends and short-term predictions estimated from surveillance data, January 1981–June 1986. *AIDS* **1**, 53–7.

Draper, N.R. and Smith, H. (1981). Applied regression analysis, (2nd edn). Wiley, New York.

van Druten, J.A.M., de Boo, Th., Jager, J.C., Heisterkamp, S.H., Coutinho, R.A., and Ruitenberg, E.J. (1986). AIDS prediction and intervention. *Lancet* **i**, 852–3.

Gonzalez, J. and Koch, M. (1986). On the role of the transients for the prognostic analysis of AIDS and the anciennity distribution of AIDS patients. *AIDS-Forsch (AIFO)* **11**, 621–30.

Heisterkamp, S.H., Jager, J.C., Downs, A.M., van Druten, J.A.M., de Boo, Th. (1988). Statistical estimation of AIDS incidence from surveillance data and the link with modelling of trends. These *Proceedings*, p. 17–25.

Kiessling, D., Stannat, S., Schedel, I., and Deicher, H. (1986). Überlegungen und Hochrechnungen zur Epidemiologie des 'Acquired Immunodeficiency Syndrome' in der Bundesrepublik Deutschland. *Infection* **14**, 217–22.

Knox, E.G. (1986). A transmission model for AIDS. *Eur. J. Epidemiol.* **2**, 165–77.

McEvoy, M. and Tillett, H.E. (1985). Some problems in the prediction of future numbers of cases of the acquired immunodeficiency syndrome in the UK. *Lancet* **ii**, 541–2.

Morgan, W.M. and Curran, J.W. (1986). Acquired immunodeficiency syndrome: current and future trends. *Public Health Reports* **101**, 459–65.

Pickering, J., Wiley, J.A., Padian, N.S., Lieb, L.E., Echenberg, D.F., and Walker, J. (1986). Modeling the incidence of acquired immunodeficiency syndrome (AIDS) in San Francisco, Los Angeles, and New York. *Mathematical Modelling* **7**, 661–88.

WHO Collaborating Centre on AIDS, Paris (1987). *AIDS surveillance in Europe report no. 13: situation by 31 March 1987*, Paris.

Acknowledgements

Data were supplied to the WHO Collaborating Centre on AIDS, Paris, by the following organizations: Conseil Supérieur de l'Hygiène Publique, Ministère de la Santé, Brussels, Belgium; Statens Serum Institute, Copenhagen, Denmark; Direction Générale de la Santé, Paris, France; Robert Koch Institute, Berlin, Federal Republic of Germany; Ministry of Health, Athens, Greece; Department of Health, Dublin, Ireland; Ministry of Health, Rome, Italy; Ministère de la Santé, Luxembourg; Staatstoezicht op de Volksgezondheid, Leidschendam, The Netherlands; Instituto Nacional de Saude, Lisbon, Portugal; Ministerio de Sanidad y Consumo, Madrid, Spain;

National Bacteriological Laboratory, Stockholm, Sweden; Office Fédéral de la Santé Publique, Berne, Switzerland; Communicable Diseases Surveillance Centre, London, UK.

This work was supported by a grant from the European Commission to the Epidemiology Subgroup of the EC Working Group on AIDS.

2

Statistical estimation of AIDS incidence from surveillance data and the link with modelling of trends

S.H. Heisterkamp, J.C. Jager, A.M. Downs, J.A.M. van Druten, and E.J. Ruitenberg

1. Introduction

Reported data on AIDS cases are rarely up to date. In Europe, for example, cases are reported to the WHO Collaborating Centre on AIDS, Paris, for up to at least 2 years following diagnosis (Downs, Ancelle, Jager, and Brunet 1987; Downs *et al.* 1988). A problem thus arises if the reported data are to be used to estimate past, present, and possibly future numbers of AIDS cases. A statistical procedure has been developed in an attempt to deal with this problem. The proposed procedure makes use of the numbers of reported cases, classified according to both period of diagnosis and period of reporting, and provides a statistically sound model-based approach to the estimation of the expected numbers of diagnosed cases, the so-called 'adjusted cases' of Downs *et al.* (1987; 1988). The estimators are shown to be related to those known from log-linear models with missing data. Since the method yields information about the variance and covariance between the adjusted cases, it becomes possible to predict future incidence using a statistically sound method provided that a suitable functional form can be chosen to model incidence trends over a sufficiently long period of time. In such an approach the trend parameters are estimated, along with the reporting-delay parameters, in a single optimization procedure, thus removing the need for explicit estimates of the adjusted case numbers. Both the frequently used exponential growth model and the logistic growth model are considered for illustrative purposes.

2. Problem

Morgan and Curran (1986) and Downs *et al.* (1987, 1988) have proposed estimates for the real numbers of cases, the so-called adjusted numbers of cases, which are then used in a regression model with time as the independent variable in order to predict future cases. However, neither method makes use of an explicitly formulated model according to which the real, but unknown,

numbers of cases are assumed to be reported. In standard statistical parametric estimation a model is assumed in order to derive efficient estimators
and associated variances and covariances. Intuitively it is clear that the
adjusted numbers of cases—the estimates for the real numbers—must have
different variances and possibly non-zero covariances. Although Downs *et
al.* (1987, 1988) and Morgan and Curran (1986) deal with the hetero-
scedasticity of the variances, the former by means of a logarithmic transformation and the latter by a Box–Cox transformation and the use of the
delta method in order to estimate the variances, the possibly non-zero covariance between the adjusted counts is neglected. Moreover, a two-stage procedure, involving the estimation of adjusted cases and the subsequent estimation of regression parameters, is likely to be less efficient then a one-stage
maximum-likelihood procedure.

3. Basic model: no trends

For each reporting period under consideration, the available data consisted
of the numbers of AIDS cases first reported in that period and diagnosed in
specified periods. We assume that for each period of diagnosis the numbers
of AIDS cases, denoted by $N_{.1}, N_{.2}, \ldots, N_{.t}$, are fixed but not observable.
We denote by n_{ij} the numbers of cases which are diagnosed in period j and
first reported in period i. The total reported incidence for period of diagnosis
j at a given time t is then given by the expression

$$n_{.j} = \sum_{i=1}^{t} n_{ij}. \tag{2.1}$$

Our basic assumptions will be that in principle all the cases could be known,
i.e. we define our sources as the ultimate, although incomplete, truth. We
also assume that all reported cases are correctly assigned, i.e. false diagnosis
or recording errors with respect to time period are neglected. Furthermore we
assume that, for a given country, reporting proportions are equal for an
equal delay between date of report and date of diagnosis. This assumption is
not really essential for the model. It could be argued, for example, that the
delay time between diagnosis and reporting could be negatively or positively
changed by directives of the authorities. It is not difficult to adapt the estimation procedure for such changes. Additional assumptions have to be made
in order to complete our parametric model. The numbers n_{ij} of first reported
cases are assumed to be Poisson distributed and statistically independent for
all i and j. This means that reporting of cases will be without clustering. Later
we shall show that this assumption could be relaxed because we condition our
distribution of first reported cases with the reported incidences. Bishop,
Fienberg, and Holland (1975) give several examples of models which measure
change in time; the model proposed here is rather simple and fits well in the

Table 2.1. Assumptions in the basic model.

$n_{ij} \approx P_0 i(\theta_{ij})$	Number of cases diagnosed in period j and first reported in period i
$\theta_{ij} = N_j p_k$	With $k = i - j$, $1 \le j \le i \le t$, $p_k > 0$, $\sum_{k}^{\infty} p_k = 1$
p_k $(k = 0, \ldots, t - 1)$	Proportion of cases of expected incidence reported with a delay of k periods
N_j	Expected incidence for the jth period of diagnosis

Table 2.2. Expected number of first reported cases in the basic model.

	Period of diagnosis						
Reporting time	81a	. . .	84a	84b	85a	85b	86a
84a	$p_6 N_{.1}$	. . .	$p_0 N_{.7}$				
84b	$p_7 N_{.1}$	. . .	$p_1 N_{.7}$	$p_0 N_{.8}$			
85a	$p_8 N_{.1}$	. . .	$p_2 N_{.7}$	$p_1 N_{.8}$	$p_0 N_{.9}$		
85b	$p_9 N_{.1}$	. . .	$p_3 N_{.7}$	$p_2 N_{.8}$	$p_1 N_{.9}$	$p_0 N_{.10}$	
86a	$p_{10} N_{.1}$	. . .	$p_4 N_{.7}$	$p_3 N_{.8}$	$p_2 N_{.9}$	$p_1 N_{.10}$	$p_0 N_{.11}$
Expected cases	$N_{.1}$	. . .	$N_{.7}$	$N_{.8}$	$N_{.9}$	$N_{.10}$	$N_{.11}$

Expected incidences are unobservable.

general framework of log-linear models and generalized linear models (McCullagh and Nelder 1983). The parameters of the Poisson distribution are then modelled according to our basic assumptions, which are summarized in Table 2.1.

The expected numbers of first reported cases are displayed in Table 2.2. As we only have observations on the reported cases the expected case numbers N_j are the parameters of interest and the reporting proportions p_k are nuisance parameters. They are estimated by fitting the basic model. This has been done using the maximum-likelihood method.

4. Maximum-likelihood estimation for the basic model

The maximum-likelihood equations are easily derived:

$$\hat{N}_j = \sum_{i=j}^{t} n_{ij} \Big/ \sum_{k=0}^{t-j} \hat{p}_k \qquad j = 1, 2 \ldots, t \tag{2.2}$$

$$\hat{p}_k = \sum_{l=1}^{t-k} n_{l+k,l} \Big/ \sum_{l=1}^{t-k} \hat{N}_j \qquad k = 0, 1, 2 \ldots, t - 1. \tag{2.3}$$

In equation (2.2) the sum in the numerator represents the reported total incidence at time t for the jth period of diagnosis, while the denominator sums over the estimated reporting proportions corresponding to this period. In equation (2.3) the summation is performed for both the numerator and the denominator parallel to the diagonal of the truncated triangular matrix in Table 2.2. The denominator represents the sum over the estimated real numbers of cases, as far as they are relevant for delay k, and the numerator represents the corresponding sum over the first reported cases with a fixed delay k.

The solutions are surprisingly straightforward and can easily be calculated using the iterative proportional fitting algorithm (Bishop *et al.* 1975). It is not possible to obtain the exact distribution of the estimators. As we require some knowledge of the variance–covariance structure of the estimators, we have to rely on the asymptotic properties of the maximum-likelihood estimators for large sample sizes (Cox and Hinkley 1974), which we consider in the next section.

5. Asymptotic variance–covariance matrix of expected incidences

The asymptotic variance–covariance matrix of the expected incidences could give us some insight into the sign and magnitude of the covariances. Owing to space restrictions we cannot give all the results of our investigation. We mention only that we have used the standard technique of computing the expectation of the Fisher information matrix (Cox and Hinkley 1974). As inversion of the resulting matrix does not give explicit solutions, inferences are made on what could be obtained from smaller matrices. The compu-tations are rather tedious, but are not really necessary in practice because standard non-linear regression algorithms provide us with estimates of this variance–covariance matrix. Our results can be summarized as follows. If the N_j are monotonically increasing, the variance of $\hat{N}_j$ increases. The covariance between N_j and N_i is positive and decreases for $k > k'$ with $k = |i - j|$.

Our second goal was to evaluate the consequences for further modelling of trends. It is known that, if a positive correlation exists between the obser-vations, the variance of the regression coefficients is inflated compared with uncorrelated observations. Therefore it is probable that the variance for prediction and estimation of future observations is much greater than the variance estimated with ordinary least squares.

One line of further work on fitting models for adjusted incidence numbers could be the use of generalized least squares by using the estimated variance–covariance matrix as a matrix of weights. In a later section of this paper a different approach will be pursued in which the estimated adjusted case numbers will no longer be needed as such.

6. Another approach: conditional estimators

Another approach to the problem of estimating the parameters involved is the use of the conditional likelihood. The problem can be reformulated as a missing-value problem: how many cases are not reported at each reporting time? To solve this we could construct a table of reported cases and leave an entry for the not yet reported cases for each period (which are missing of course). For each period j we then have a multinomial distribution of reported and not yet reported cases with unknown parameters p_0 to p_{i-j} and N_j. Each of the not yet reported cases has a multinomial probability $1-\Sigma p$ of being reported. This distribution can be constructed from the independent Poisson distributions by conditioning on the total numbers of cases that can be reported in each period of time (Bishop *et al.* 1975). We can then write the likelihood function as the product of two likelihoods: the binomial likelihood function of the non-reported cases and the conditional multinomial likelihood function of the cases which have already been reported. The total likelihood is then the product of the above mentioned likelihood functions for all periods of diagnosis. It can be shown that in our case the conditional solution is exactly the same as the unconditional solution. According to Bishop *et al.* (1975) conditional and unconditional estimators are generally not the same. However, asymptotically they both have the same multivariate normal distribution. As both methods yield the same estimators, we are encouraged in pursuing this line of thought.

7. Extending the basic model: modelling trends

Until now it has been assumed that there is a positive probability of reporting a case after an infinite time delay, but this does not seem to be very realistic. For this reason a further restriction is imposed on the statistical model we have used so far. We assume for each period of diagnosis that after a certain delay T, which can be chosen arbitrarily, no new cases are reported, i.e. we put

$$\sum_{k=0}^{T} p_k = 1. \tag{2.4}$$

This condition changes the likelihood equations, since the derivatives with respect to the independent parameters p_k ($k = 0,1, \ldots, T-1$) are changed. The likelihood equations are now less straightforward than those presented in equations (2.2) and (2.3), and the solutions are not presented here. In fact we now obtain, at least numerically, the same estimates as those given by Downs *et al.* (1987, 1988).

A further modification had to be made before the procedure could be used with data reported to WHO, Paris, since reporting began only in 1984. Only aggregated data (the current reported incidences) were available at the first reporting time. This problem was solved by assuming that the same reporting-delay pattern would have existed before 1984. Thus, for each diagnostic period, the number of cases expected to be reported in the first 6 months of 1984 is the sum of the cases expected to have been reported at earlier times. This further complicates the maximum-likelihood equations.

Finally we consider the possible modelling of trends. We make no attempt here to discuss which particular model should be chosen. It is clear that, as the AIDS epidemic is rather new, statistical evidence alone is not enough to discriminate between different models for trends. The models to be considered have to be derived by mathematical epidemiological considerations (van Druten, de Boo, Jager, Heisterkamp, Coutinho, and Ruitenberg 1986; May and Anderson 1987). Furthermore, it is not important whether the model is formulated as an explicit function or is more implicit (see, for example, Brookmeyer and Gail 1986). However, whatever model is chosen, it is of great importance to estimate its parameters with efficient statistical techniques in order to obtain appropriate confidence limits (via, for example, the variance–covariance matrix).

Table 2.3.   Models for the expected incidences.

Model expectations	$N_j = f(t_j, \theta)$
Exponential model	$f(t, \alpha, \beta) = \alpha e^{\beta} t$
Integrated logistic	$f(t, \alpha, \beta, \psi) = \psi \ln \left\{ \dfrac{e^{\beta(t-\alpha)} + 1}{e^{\beta(t-\alpha)} e^{-\beta} + 1} \right\}$

The function chosen to model the expected incidence N_j (Table 2.3) replaces each N_j in Table 2.2. This reduces considerably the number of parameters of the model; for example, the t parameters N_j are replaced by two parameters in the exponential model or by three parameters in the integrated logistic model. In fact it is no longer necessary to estimate explicitly the 'adjusted cases' N_j. The resulting maximum-likelihood equations can be solved only by numerical methods. We have used the Genstat statistical programming language (Alvey, *et al.* 1983) to do this.

8. Results for The Netherlands

For illustration, we give some results for The Netherlands. Observed and fitted values and estimated incidence are given for the basic model (i.e. the model without a trend) in Table 2.4. Parameter estimates for the basic model, the exponential model, and the integrated logistic model are given in Table 2.5. Note that in fact we should have given fitted values and reporting proportions for each of the different models. One advantage of the proposed

Table 2.4. Basic model applied to data for The Netherlands: observed and fitted values.

Reporting time	Period of diagnosis								
	82a	82b	83a	83b	84a	84b	85a	85b	86a
84a	(1)	(2)	(6)	(7)	5				
Fitted	1	2	5.7	8.1	4.4				
84b			0	1	1	19			
Fitted			0.3	0.5	1.0	17.5			
85a				1	0	4	19		
Fitted				0.4	0.4	4.1	21.3		
85b					0	0	6	26	
Fitted					0.3	1.4	4.9	25.1	
86a						1	3	5	39
Fitted						1.1	1.7	5.8	39
TOTAL	1	2	6	9	6	24	28	31	39
EXPECTED	1	2	6	9	6	24	29.3	34.6	53.6

Table 2.5. Parameter estimates for various models in The Netherlands.

		Deviance	DF
Basic model expected incidences	1 2 6 9 6 24 29.3 34.6 53.6	7.343	9
Rep. proportions	0.73 0.17 0.06 0.04		
Exponential model		15.840	16
a 2.18	SE 0.60		
b 0.410	SE 0.045		
Doubling time	10 months		
Integrated logistic (incidences)		14.165	15
a 7.61	SE 1.98		
b 0.566	SE 0.13		
c 143.6	SE 113		

estimation procedure is the possibility of assessing the goodness of fit. We chose the deviance as the measure of goodness of fit (Nelder and Wedderburn 1972; McCullagh and Nelder 1983). Although it is questionable whether the deviance is χ^2 distributed (McCullagh and Nelder 1983), it gives an important clue as to whether a model fits or not. From the difference in deviance between the exponential model and the integrated logistic model it is not evident that the latter fit is better. The number of degrees of freedom for the deviance is calculated as the difference between the number of observations involved and the number of estimated parameters, including the $T-1$ reporting proportions. Note that zero n_{ij} with $i-j > T$ are the so-called 'structural zeros' (Bishop *et al.* 1975) and are not regarded as observations.

9. Discussion and conclusions

A statistical estimation procedure has been developed using the maximum-likelihood method to estimate the expected incidence of AIDS cases from the reported incidence in the absence of a model for trend. If a suitable function can be chosen, parameters can be estimated in an efficient one-stage procedure without actually using the 'adjusted cases'. However, it should be remembered that the validity of the projections made outside the observed time range will depend heavily on the appropriateness of the model in describing the future course of the epidemic. There is considerable evidence that doubling times are increasing, implying that the exponential model is not applicable for future predictions. However, there is no obvious justification, at the present time, for preferring any one of several possible alternatives. A more pragmatic approach which attempts to make some allowance for the expected departure from exponential growth by making use of time windows has therefore been adopted by Downs *et al.* (1987, 1988). The procedure used here is flexible enough to allow for different types of function in the modelling of trends. We believe that a sound statistical procedure is essential for estimating parameters and confidence limits for future incidence, given an epidemiological model based on information about the spread of the disease. The assessment of a model, whether using an explicit function or a more implicitly defined function (Brookmeyer and Gail 1986), can only be done by statistical means, and projections for the future are always based on the assumption of *ceteris paribus*.

References

Alvey, N.G., Banfield, C.F., Baxter, R.I., Gower, J.C., Krzanowski, W.J., Lane, P.W., Leech, P.W., Nelder, J.A., Payne, R.W., Phelps, K.M., Rogers, C.E., Ross, G.J.S., Simpson, H.R., Todd, A.D., Tunnicliffe-Wilson, G., Wedderburn, R.W.M., White, R.P., and Wilkinson, G.N. (1983). *Genstat. A general statistical program*. Numerical Algorithms Group, Oxford.

Bishop, Y.M.M., Fienberg, S.E., and Holland, P.W. (1975). *Discrete multivariate analysis: Theory and practice*. MIT Press, Cambridge, Mass.

Brookmeyer, R. and Gail, M.H. (1986). Minimum size of the acquired immuno-deficiency syndrome (AIDS) epidemic in the United States. *Lancet* **ii**, 1320-2.

Cox, D.R. and Hinkley, D.V. (1974). *Theoretical statistics*. Chapman and Hall, London.

Downs, A.M., Ancelle, R.A., Jager, J.C., Heisterkamp, S.H., van Druten,

J.A.M., Ruitenberg, E.J., and Brunet, J.-B. (1988). The statistical estimation, from routine surveillance data, of past, present and future trends in AIDS incidence in Europe. These *Proceedings*, pp. 1-16.

Downs, A.M., Ancelle R.A., Jager J.C. and Brunet, J.-B. (1987). AIDS in Europe: current trends and short-term predictions estimated from surveillance data, January 1981-June 1986. *AIDS* **1**, 53-57.

van Druten, J.A.M., de Boo, Th., Jager, J.C., Heisterkamp, S.H., Coutinho, R.A., and Ruitenberg, E.J. (1986). AIDS Prediction and Intervention. *Lancet* **i**, 852-3.

May, R.M. and Anderson, R.M. (1987). Transmission dynamics of HIV infection. *Nature, London* **326**, 137-42.

McCullagh, P. and Nelder, J.A. (1983). *Generalized linear models*. Chapman and Hall, London.

Morgan, W.M. and Curran, J.W. (1986). Acquired immunodeficiency syndrome: current and future trends. *Public Health Reports* **101**, 459-65.

Nelder, J.A. and Wedderburn, R.W.M. (1972). Generalized linear models. *Journal of the Royal Statistical Society A* **135**, 370-84.

3

Observations from the UK epidemic

H.E. Tillett

---

1. Introduction

Cases of AIDS diagnosed in the UK are reported on a voluntary basis to the Communicable Disease Surveillance Centre (CDSC) and to the Communicable Diseases (Scotland) Unit. Study of these data has suggested that short-term predictions based on the standard statistical model can be presented in a more helpful way, that routine data can be used to make a rough estimation of incubation periods, and that longer-term predictions based on these observations can demonstrate hypothetically the effects of intervention strategies.

2. Short-term predictions

In common with other countries the curve in the early years of the AIDS epidemic in the UK has been essentially log-linear in shape. Projections from such a regression analysis have been published (Tillett and McEvoy 1986) and are expected to be valid until about 1988, but more information is needed before longer-term predictions should be attempted. Nevertheless, it is felt that the methodology and presentation of these short-term predictions can be improved.

The published regression and predictions have been made using numbers of cases by year of presentation for medical advice. However, the cases may not be reported for some considerable time afterwards—about one-fifth of cases have already died when the report form is received. Some delays are inevitable, and it is far more important to the surveillance scheme that the reporting should be as complete as possible than that it should be immediate.

Previous analyses have omitted data from recent time periods because numbers were known to be incomplete: thus much information was wasted. It is planned instead to analyse by date of report, which will always be a consistent data set (once duplicate reports have been eliminated). However, health care planners wish to know how many new cases to expect in the near future. Therefore adjustments will have to be made to the new predictions by allowing for the probable period between onset and reporting. For onset we shall in future use the date at which the case fulfils the WHO–CDC case definition in order to be consistent with other countries. These time intervals

26

are currently being studied. The statistical model will also take into account the effect of 'transients' (Gonzalez and Koch 1986, 1987)—the anomalies due to the over-representation of cases with short incubation periods in the early part of the epidemic—thus the early rate of increase in cases will be greater than the infection rate and, later in the epidemic, there will be a compensating artificial slowing down.

3. Incubation period

The routine data-reporting systems, including that of laboratory reports of HIV-positive patients, can be used to estimate possible incubation periods for AIDS in different risk groups. These estimates will not be as reliable as those given by cohort studies.

In the UK the greatest numbers of AIDS cases have been in homosexuals. This is the only risk group for which this method of estimating possible minimum incubation period has been done. So far, numbers in other risk groups are too few. In 1985 there were 485 HIV-positive patients reported by laboratories to CDSC who were stated to be homosexuals. Clinical information was received for about 70 per cent of the patients. These included 125 who were asymptomatic and whose median age at the time of testing was 28 years. 219 patients were reported with pre-AIDS symptoms (such as fever, diarrhoea, weight loss, or lymphadenopathy) and their median age was 31 years. The reporting scheme for clinical AIDS in the UK had produced 139 cases in homosexuals with onset during 1985 and reported by August 1986. Their median age was 36 years.

These data suggest that among homosexuals the time interval between asymptomatic antibody positivity and onset of AIDS could be of the order of 8 years. This estimate is likely to err on the low side since it is not known how long the asymptomatic patients had been antibody positive.

4. Hypothetical heterosexual epidemic and intervention

If there is a heterosexually spread epidemic in the UK, it is possible that, in common with other epidemics, the early years will see an exponential spread of infection doubling time may be of the order of 1 year. (For homosexual cases in the UK it is currently estimated to be 10 months.) The means incubation period might be similar to that of homosexually spread AIDS. If the incubation period is dose related, it might be even longer.

Table 3.1 shows a hypothetical exponential epidemic constructed with a doubling time of 1 year and an incubation period for AIDS averaging 8 years. The distribution of incubation periods is unknown but has been assumed here to follow a gamma distribution. The choice of distribution is not crucial since the aim is to demonstrate when the first cases might develop.

Table 3.1.   Hypothetical heterosexually spread epidemic.

| Year | New fatal HIV infections† | AIDS cases (onset)‡ | Intervention in year 11 (20 per cent effective) | | |
			New fatal HIV infections§	Infection 'prevented' per year	Cumulative infections 'prevented'
0	1				
1	2				
2	4				
3	8				
4	16				
5	32				
6	64	1			
7	128	2			
8	256	4			
9	512	8			
10	1024	15			
11	2048	30	2048		
12	4096	61	3649	447	447
13	8192	121	6502	1690	2137
14	16384	243	11585	4799	6936
15	32768	485	20646	12122	19058
16	65536	970	36786	28750	47808

†Infections that will lead to AIDS (assumed to be a constant proportion of the total infections).
‡Assuming a gamma distribution for incubation periods, with mean and variance of 8 years; thus some cases develop before the mean period has elapsed.
§That is lengthening the doubling time from 12 to 14.4 months.

Bearing in mind that there can be delay in reporting, the epidemic might become apparent in about year 10. Introducing intervention schemes in year 11 which slow down the rate of spread by just 20 per cent can prevent or delay many thousands of cases. Thus general public education schemes would seem to be well worthwhile and effectively 'buy' time while more specifically targeted prevention strategies are discussed and planned, and while resources are put into developing treatment and vaccines.

5. Summary

Recent statistical studies of AIDS cases in the UK (England, Wales, Scotland, and Northern Ireland) have raised three points.

Firstly, short-term predictions of the epidemic curve are easier to make from numbers of cases using date of report rather than date of onset.

However, health care planners require information on probable numbers of new cases by year of onset, and adjustments must be made to allow for the time intervals between onset and report. The effect of transients has also been considered.

Secondly, looking at routine data, the median age of HIV-positive homosexual men, reported by laboratories, has been 28 years for those stated to be asymptomatic. The median age at onset of male homosexual cases of AIDS has been 36 years, which suggests that the incubation period in this risk group may be of the order of 8 years.

Thirdly, a hypothetical epidemic of heterosexually acquired AIDS has been constructed also with a mean incubation period of 8 years. It can be shown that an intervention programme introduced when the first few AIDS cases have been reported—even if it is only partially successful in slowing down the rate of spread—can prevent large numbers of fatal cases.

References

Gonzalez, J.J. and Koch, M.G. (1986). On the role of the transients for the prognostic analysis of AIDS. *AIDS-Forschung (AIFO)* **11**, 621–30.

Gonzalez, J.J. and Koch, M.G. (1987). On the role of 'transients' (biasing transitional effects) for the prognostic analysis of the AIDS epidemic. *American Journal of Epidemiology* **126**, 985–1005.

Tillett, H.E. and McEvoy, M. (1986) Reassessment of predicted numbers of AIDS cases in the UK. *Lancet* **ii**, 1104.

4

Predicting the AIDS epidemic from trends elsewhere

S.C. Richardson, C. Caroni, and G. Papaevangelou

1. Introduction

The first AIDS case in Greece occurred at the end of 1983, and the total had reached 32 by the end of 1986. From this small number of cases in a short period of time, can we make good numerical predictions of the course of the epidemic, in the next year at least? The answer seems to be 'no' if we follow the simple methodology of fitting a curve to the historical data and extrapolating forward. This approach has been applied to predict AIDS cases in other countries,[1-3] and it is always pointed out that there are many uncertainties in these predictions, not only in the sense that they carry large standard errors but also in whether or not the stability of the various factors involved is sufficient to permit extrapolation.[1,4,5] In fact there is no evidence that the shape of the AIDS epidemic curve can change very quickly, so that extrapolation is valid if we restrict ourselves to a suitably short period of time, such as 1 year. We therefore concentrate on the statistical aspects of prediction. The standard errors for Greece will indeed be very large, as we see in Section 2 where this prediction exercise is carried out. How can they be reduced? Only by having more information, and the only possibility—if we are to make predictions now and not simply wait to accumulate more data for Greece—is to see if we can exploit data from other countries, particularly those in which the epidemic has advanced further than it has as yet in Greece. The need to employ methodology which does not simply use the data from one country or area in isolation from others is the point we wish to emphasize.

2. Forecasts for Greece

A method used elsewhere[1,3] involves fitting a straight line to the logarithm of the numbers of cases occuring in suitable intervals of time, say 6 months. Table 4.1 shows the data for Greece together with fitted values and predictions from the regression equation

$$\ln (\text{cases}) = \underset{(0.278)}{0.346} + \underset{(0.071)}{0.345}\, t \qquad t = 1 \ldots 6$$

Table 4.1. Predictions of AIDS cases in Greece from regression of the logarithm of number of cases against time.

Period	Cases		Residual†	Predicted
	Observed	Fitted		
− 6.84	2	2.0	0.01	—
7.84–12.84	4	2.8	1.17	—
1.85– 6.85	3	4.0	− 0.95	—
7.85–12.85	4	5.6	− 1.14	—
1.86– 6.86	9	7.9	0.42	—
7.86–12.86‡	13	11.2	0.50	—
1.87– 6.87	—	—	—	15.8
				(5.1, 49.1)§
7.87–12.87	—	—	—	22.4
				(6.3, 79.0)

†Internally Studentized residual.
‡Three cases confirmed on 5.1.87 are included in 1986.
§95 per cent confidence interval.

(R^2 = 0.854 and the standard error is 0.298). The doubling time of the epidemic is estimated at 12.1 months (95 per cent confidence interval, 7.9–25.4 months). The predicted total of new cases for 1987 is 38.

Variations of this simple methodology include fitting a quadratic in time to the number of cases.[2] This predicts 44 new cases for 1987: 18.6 (95 per cent confidence interval, 13.0–24.3) in the first half of the year and 25.5 (19.2–31.8) in the second half. These intervals are much shorter than for the other curve and both curves fit adequately according to standard regression diagnostics, so at this stage the quadratic regression seems to be preferable for use with our data. However, the quadratic does not seem to be applicable in other countries beyond this early stage of the epidemic.

While these predictions can be of some use (they at least reassure the planners that the need for 1987 is for facilities for under 100 cases), they cannot hope to achieve high precision, and tinkering with the methodology will not lead to radical improvement. However, a different approach might produce benefits. In fact we would say from a logical point of view that there is a definite need for a different approach. The above fitting exercise would be precisely the same if AIDS were an isolated phenomenon which existed nowhere except in Greece and we had no idea whether the size of the problem would continue to increase or whether the disease would shortly disappear again. In reality, the latter possibility can be excluded because external and internal evidence point to continued development of the epidemic. We know from the experience of other countries that the disease can be expected to increase with a regression coefficient of around 0.4 for the logarithm of cases against time,[3] while locally we know that there are at least 200 HIV carriers, at least some of whom will develop the disease sooner or later. This prior information should be incorporated into the analysis in some way. This could be done by carrying out a fully Bayesian analysis, defining prior distributions for the regression parameters to represent the knowledge accumulated from elsewhere and deriving posterior distributions from which predictions can be obtained. For illustration, however, we have chosen simply to use the mixed estimation procedure of Theil and Goldberger.[6] In this, we specify a range in which the regression slope is assumed to lie. We have chosen 0.3–0.6, which covers the values calculated for most European countries in different periods by Downs, Ancelle, Jager, and Brunet,[3] with the notable exception of Italy.

The revised estimate of the regression slope (for the log-linear regression) becomes 0.388 (standard error, 0.055). The estimated doubling time is thus 10.7 months (7.7–17.7 months). The length of this interval is 43 per cent shorter than that given above, which is a considerable gain for assuming no more than that the epidemic in Greece will increase at a rate within the range of other European countries. The corresponding number of new cases in 1987 is now put at 41, and so the point prediction has not changed very much.

3. Fitting the same model to different countries

It is often remarked that the growth of the AIDS epidemic is very similar from place to place. Essentially, we have used this fact in assuming above that Greece's growth rate will be similar to rates experienced in nearby countries. But can we go further and assume equal growth rates? We would then have an even better means of numerical prediction.

Predictions for the UK from the experience of the USA were derived in a rough way by Mortimer,[5] who assumed a lag of 3 years between the epidemics in the two countries and also assumed that the number of cases at equivalent times should be proportional to the populations of the countries. The first assumption is open to improvement by statistical estimation. The second is very dubious. We are only talking about the early stages of an epidemic, in which the spread is largely confined to particular high risk groups whose size need not be simply proportional to the country's total population. Therefore, if a proportionality is admitted, the sizes of the high risk groups are the relevant quantities. Generally the data are sufficient only for a guess at these. However, a constant of proportionality could, like the lag, be estimated statistically in a suitable model.

In this section, we carry out statistical analyses of the development of the epidemic in groups of states or countries. If we fail to find close similarity in detail, this makes it unlikely that it is appropriate to apply the exact experience of other countries to make predictions for Greece.

The curve fitted to the data is the Gompertz growth curve

$$\ln(N_t) = \alpha - \beta\rho^t,$$

with $\rho < 1$, where N_t is the total number of cases at the time period t. This was chosen for convenience from among the many available curves which seem to give reasonably good descriptions of the growth of the epidemic. As we are only talking about the early stages of the epidemic, it does not matter that in the long run the Gompertz curve is an implausible description. It has the advantage over the log-linear regression that it gives a declining rate of increase, which agrees with observation, rather than a constant rate. Curves of the general modified exponential family to which the Gompertz curve belongs also have the advantage that models for different areas with a time lag are easily related. Specifically, if Y_{it} is the log count in area i at time t and log counts in area j are proportional to those occurring τ time periods earlier in area i, so that

$$Y_{j,t+\tau} = \lambda Y_{it},$$

or, assuming that parameters α and β vary between areas but the growth parameter ρ is common

$$\alpha_j - \beta_j\rho^{t+\tau} = \lambda(\alpha_i - \beta_i\rho^t),$$

then

$$\frac{\alpha_j}{\alpha_i} = \frac{\beta_j\rho^\tau}{\beta_i} = \lambda.$$

Thus the lag τ can be estimated by obtaining estimates $\{\alpha_i, \beta_i\}$ and ρ and then solving

$$\tau \ln \rho = \ln \left(\frac{\beta_i\alpha_j}{\beta_j\alpha_i} \right).$$

Thus the time lag is not an explicit feature of the model as fitted but rather an interpretation of the differences between estimates. In presenting the results, we shall take one area—the one where the epidemic developed first—as the reference and obtain an estimated lag τ and constant of proportionality λ for each other area in relation to it.

The model was fitted first, for illustration, to quarterly data for eight major states of the USA, and gave the estimated lags and proportions shown in Table 4.2. Fitting was by ordinary least squares, directly minimizing the residual sum of squares over $\alpha_1, \ldots, \alpha_8, \beta_1, \ldots, \beta_8, \rho$ using the subroutine ZXSSQ from the IMSL library. The model does not fit in the statistical sense (the F ratio for the increase in residual sum of squares over the eight separate models with unconstrained ρ is 44.7 on 7 and 136 degrees of freedom, $p < 0.001$) and no doubt should be improved, at least by using some form

Table 4.2.   Analysis for eight USA states: estimated lags and constants of proportionality relative to New York.

State	CA	FL	MA	IL	NJ	PA	TX
Lag (months)	11.1	13.7	17.5	18.4	19.6	22.0	22.9
Proportionality	1.05	0.91	0.70	0.74	0.98	0.80	0.96

Data: quarterly totals, 1.1.80–31.3.85.

of weighting, but the graph in Fig. 4.1 does enable us to see important features of the data. In this figure the counts for California, Texas, and Pennsylvania are plotted advanced by the appropriate number of time periods and multiplied by the appropriate proportion, along with the counts for New York. Curves for the other states are omitted for clarity: Florida and New Jersey fall very close to Texas, and the others are close to Pennsylvania.

The same model was next fitted to Europe. The data used were 6-monthly totals for all countries with more than 50 cases up to July 1986, excluding Belgium and Italy (generally regarded as special cases, as the former has a majority of Africans among its cases and the latter shows an exceptionally rapid spread of the disease among intravenous drug abusers) and including Greece. In place of the reported numbers we used figures adjusted for reporting delays, kindly supplied by Dr A.M. Downs of the WHO Colla-

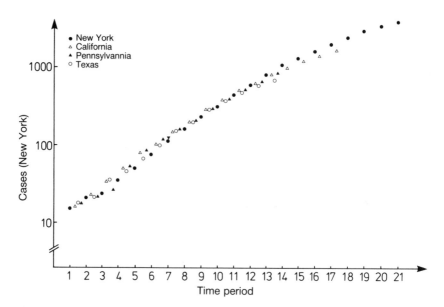

Fig. 4.1.   Counts for California, Texas, Pennsylvania, and New York (for explanation see text).

Table 4.3. Analysis for nine European countries: estimated lags and constants of proportionality relative to France.

Country	UK	Switz	Denmark	FRG	Spain	Neth	Sweden	Greece
Lag (months)	9.4	15.5	19.1	26.4	33.4	34.6	40.1	53.5
Proportionality	1.00	0.83	0.81	1.27	1.16	1.16	0.98	1.00

borating Centre, Paris. Lags estimated relative to France are shown in Table 4.3. The fit was again poor in comparison with separate models for each country and was worst for the FRG and The Netherlands, where the latest figures are well below those expected despite the adjustment for reporting delays. Although we remarked in Section 1 that the epidemic curve could not change fast enough to invalidate short-term predictions, it is possible that reporting processes (including willingness to report as well as the actual systems) can change with relatively abrupt effects. The fit for Greece, however, was relatively good. The predicted number for Greece for the second half of 1986 was 15.2 compared with the 13 actually occurring. The predicted number for 1987 was 59. Notice that this is substantially above the estimates derived above. This is because the model fitted here employs a common growth parameter, and the contribution of Greece to its estimation is swamped by the contributions of other countries with generally higher rates.

In case it should be thought that the estimated constants of proportionality have rather unusual values in Table 4.3, it should be noted that they do *not* have an interpretation in terms of the ratio of population sizes, since our curves are fitted to the logarithms of counts and not to the counts themselves. These constants are only descriptive and are introduced with the purpose of improving the fits of the curves. The present exercise is curve fitting, not modelling.

We conclude that the approach briefly investigated here offers little for predictive purposes. The assumption of equal growth rates is inadequate, even though approximate equality is a striking feature for simple description of the AIDS epidemic. Different places may follow extremely similar paths, but the right places must be chosen and we would only know with hindsight whether the predictions for one area from the history of another were based on a correct choice or not.

4. Discussion

Our results in the previous sections indicate that there are substantial benefits to be obtained by incorporating extra information into the estimation for countries where the epidemic is still in its early stage so that little local information is yet available. This cannot be pushed too far, however; the imposition of equal growth rates, for example, seems to be statistically invalid as a general procedure, although it may be applicable in particular cases. The obvious direction for further investigation is to study models where growth rates are not equal but are to some degree linked, in other words a random-coefficients model. There is a substantial literature on this, including extensions for non-linear curves.[7]

As particular predictions for Greece are of ephemeral interest, the methodological message is the major point of our presentation. Despite the reluctance of many investigators to accept that quantitative prediction is a proper activity in the present state of epidemiological knowledge of AIDS, many of us are pressed to provide numerical forecasts. Given that requirement, the predictions should be the best possible, which means, when there is little local information, that the substantial body of external information must be exploited. The same idea is also useful in the analysis of the spread of the epidemic to new cities or regions of a country where it has already made substantial progress elsewhere.

5. Summary

If predictions of numbers of AIDS cases are to be made, logic demands that the considerable amount of prior information available from the experience of other countries should be incorporated into the analysis. The advantage of doing this is illustrated for simple regression predictions of the number of cases in Greece in 1987. A major reduction in the length of confidence intervals follows, compared with the ordinary prediction using only the present meagre data for this country. A further model investigated imposes the requirement of an equal growth parameter in each of the areas included in the analysis. Although this gives visually a striking impression of nearly equal development of the epidemic in different places, in statistical terms it seems to be too strong a requirement and not suitable for use in prediction.

References

1. McEvoy, M. and Tillett H.E. (1985). Some problems in the prediction of future numbers of cases of the acquired immunodeficiency syndrome in the UK. *Lancet* ii, 541-2.
2. Artalejo, F.R., Albero, M.J.M., Alvarez, F.V., Laguarta, A.B., and Caballero J.G. (1986). Predicting AIDS cases. *Lancet* i, 378.
3. Downs, A.M., Ancelle, R.A., Jager, J.C., and Brunet, J.-B. (1987). AIDS in Europe: current trends and short-term predictions estimated from surveillance data, January 1981-June 1986. *AIDS* 1, 53-7.
4. McEvoy, M. and Tillett, H.E. (1986). AIDS for all by the year 2000? *British Medical Journal*. **290**, 463.

5. Mortimer, P. (1985). Estimating AIDS in the UK. *Lancet* **ii**, 1065.
6. Kmenta, J. (1971). *Elements of econometrics*. McGraw-Hill, New York.
7. Cook, N.R. and Ware, J.H. (1983). Design and analysis methods for longitudinal research. *Annual Reviews of Public Health* **4**, 1–23.

5

Modelling the incidence of AIDS in New York, Los Angeles, and San Francisco

J. Pickering, J.A. Wiley, L.E. Lieb, J. Walker, and
G.W. Rutherford

1. Introduction

In 1986, an epidemic model of the population dynamics of AIDS was published (Pickering, Wiley, Padian, Lieb, Echenberg, and Walker 1986). The primary assumptions of this model are that AIDS can be modelled as a sexually transmitted disease and that the transmission rates of the agents responsible for AIDS respond as does gonorrhoea to changes in sexual behaviour. Here we update the model and analyse the incidence of AIDS in New York, San Francisco, and Los Angeles.

2. Incidence of AIDS

By June 1987 over 36 000 cases of AIDS in the United States had been reported to the Centers for Disease Control (CDC), Atlanta. Of these cases, nearly half were reported from New York, San Francisco, and Los Angeles—the three locations that continue to report the highest number of cases.

Figures 5.1–5.3 present the monthly incidence of AIDS in New York City, San Francisco County, and Los Angeles County respectively. These cases were those reported to the respective health departments by 23 July 1987, 30 June 1987, and 30 June 1987. While the health departments are likely to adopt a broader definition of AIDS cases in the near future, the cases presented meet the CDC's surveillance definition (Staff Report 1983, 1985) and are comparable across cities. Because all AIDS cases are not recognized as such, there is under-reporting of cases. The level of this bias may differ by location. New York City, for example, recently experienced an increase in the number of tuberculosis cases, up to 600 of which may be opportunistic infections that are part of the AIDS outbreak but which are not included as AIDS cases (Drucker 1987).

The figures present the majority of the cases from each regional population. Most notably, they do not include cases from eastern New Jersey in the

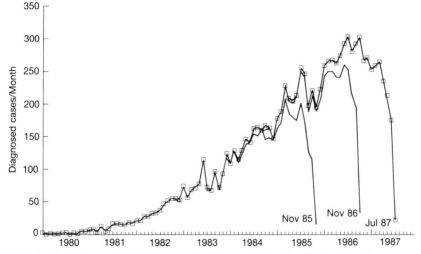

Fig. 5.1.   Incidence of AIDS by month of diagnosis for New York City. The squares represent 10 730 cases reported by 23 July 1987, to the City of New York Department of Health. The two lower lines show the cases that had been reported by 20 November 1986, and by 19 November 1985. They illustrate the magnitude of the respective time lags from when cases were diagnosed to when they were reported to the health department. Hence the most recent data for the months after October 1986, do not necessarily indicate that the epidemic is levelling off.

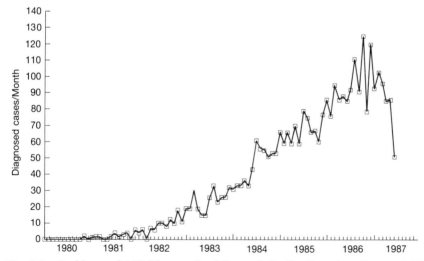

Fig. 5.2.   Incidence of AIDS by month of diagnosis for San Francisco County. 3402 cases reported by 30 June 1987 to the City and County of San Francisco Department of Public Health are included. It should not be concluded that the most recent data necessarily indicate a levelling off in the epidemic's course (see text and Fig. 5.1).

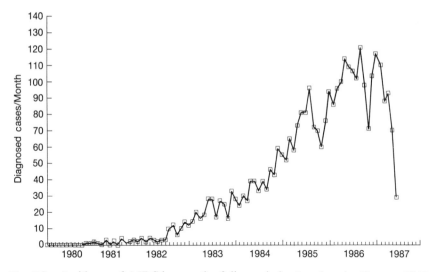

Fig. 5.3. Incidence of AIDS by month of diagnosis for Los Angeles County. 3340 cases reported by 30 June 1987 to the County of Los Angeles Department of Health Services are included. The most recent data do not necessarily indicate that the epidemic is levelling off (see text and Fig. 5.1).

case of New York, Alameda County in the case of San Francisco, and Orange County in the case of Los Angeles. San Francisco, for example, reports over 80 per cent of the cases from the Bay Area—San Francisco, Alameda, San Mateo, Contra Costa, and Marin Counties.

The figures present the cases by month of diagnosis. By analysing cases by time of diagnosis, we factor out differences in reporting lags. Considering cases by the onset of symptoms might be preferable but would be difficult, in part because of the many and varied courses manifested by the syndrome.

While the average time lag from case diagnosis to reporting to the CDC is about 4 months, (Morgan 1987), this lag creates a considerable caveat for modellers of the epidemic. It is primarily reflected in the most recent months and gives an artificial impression that the epidemic is levelling off. In Fig. 5.1 the New York cases reported by 23 July 1987 are compared with those reported by 20 November 1986 and by 19 November 1985. In retrospect, we conclude that a model that fitted the 10 most recent months of data on 20 November 1986 (i.e. those after January 1986) would have tended to underestimate the epidemic's course. On 19 November 1985 the lag was even longer, with the 16 most recent data at that time underestimating eventual values. Thus Fig. 5.1 illustrates that the lag is not constant. Because we cannot assume that the lag will be constant in the future, we do not attempt to make adjustments for it. Instead, in the following analysis, we simply do not fit data after March 1986.

Finally, Moss *et al.* (1985) suggest that some of the variance in the time when AIDS cases are diagnosed is probably not biological in origin. In particular, news media coverage may influence when individuals seek medical help and are diagnosed. For example, all three locations show a decline in the number of cases in the last four months of 1985. We model the data strictly from a biological perspective and warn that our conclusions depend on the assumption that any periodicity in the data is predominantly biological in nature.

3. Changes in sexual behaviour

Since the first reports of AIDS in mid-1981, homosexual men have changed their behaviour considerably. Declines in activities likely to transmit HIV —the infectious agent underlying AIDS—are documented by surveys of the sexual behaviour reported by homosexual men in San Francisco (McKusick, Horstman, and Coates 1985; Pickett, Bart, Bye, and Amory 1985; Werdegar, O'Malley, Bodecker, Hessol, and Echenberg 1987), New York (Martin 1987), and other metropolitan areas (Golubjatnikov, Pfister, and Tillotson 1983; Fox, Ostrow, Valdisseri, Van Raden, Visscher, and Polk 1987).

In order to predict the long-term course of the AIDS epidemic, it is necessary to understand the impact of behavioural changes on the spread of HIV. This is not a simple task to perform from survey data alone. Surveys provide data on trends in their respondents' sexual activity but generally do not provide information on the mixing among individuals with different numbers of partners. It is one thing to ask an individual how many sexual partners he or she has had. It is another to ask how many partners his or her partners have had.

Theoretically, it is necessary to consider the distribution in the number of partners individuals have and how individuals select partners as a function of partner number. For example, do individuals with many partners generally have partners with many partners? The models of Hethcote and Yorke (1984) demonstrate the potential importance of core individuals—those with a high turnover in partners—in spreading gonorrhoea. Similarly, the spread of HIV is likely to depend on the population's level of heterogeneity in sexual activity. May and Anderson (1987) argue that individuals with many new sexual partners per unit of time play a disproportionately high role in spreading the virus. They suggest that the effective measure of the number of new partners per unit time is not the mean of the distribution but the mean plus the ratio of variance to mean. In estimating HIV's infectivity, Grant, Wiley, and Winkelstein (1987) use two alternative bonding models: one assumes simple random bonding and the other assumes random bonding stratified by number of partners. The results of the two models differ but not significantly.

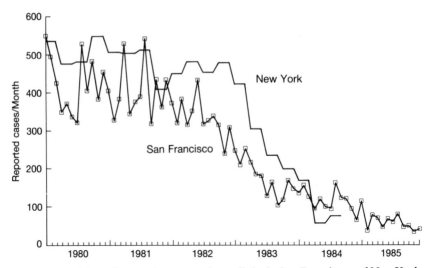

Fig. 5.4.   Anal/rectal gonorrhoea cases from clinics in San Francisco and New York. The San Francisco data are those reported by Pickering *et al.* (1986). The New York data are based on quarterly data kindly provided by Alan Kristal, formerly with the City of New York Department of Health.

The change in the behaviour of homosexual men has had an impact on other sexually transmitted diseases. The number of male anal/rectal gonorrhoea cases has declined in Denver, CO (Judson 1983), New York (Schultz, Friedman, Kristal, and Senser 1984), and San Francisco (Pickering *et al.* 1986). Given the difficulty of documenting and modelling trends in sexual contact rates with survey data, we use gonorrhoea cases as an indirect index of the behavioural changes that have occurred. Figure 5.4 shows the number of anal/rectal gonorrhoea cases at sexually transmitted disease clinics in San Fran cisco and New York. If it is assumed that cure rates remained constant, these data suggest that behaviour changed earlier in San Francisco than in New York. In addition to safer sexual behaviour, increased awareness and screening of asymptomatic gonorrhoea cases may also have contributed to the decline. In modelling Los Angeles, we use the gonorrhoea data from San Francisco.

4. Outline of the model

The following equation is derived by Pickering *et al.* (1986) and attempts to characterize the underlying factors affecting the incidence of AIDS. It considers the factors that we presume are important based on epidemic theory and the known biology of AIDS:

$$D_t \approx \frac{\kappa}{1 - \kappa_g R'_{t-\delta}} \left(\sum_{i=t-\delta+\sigma}^{t-\delta+\mu} D_i \right) \left(1 - \kappa_a \sum_{i=0}^{t-1} D_i \right)$$

For month t, we let D_t be the number of AIDS cases diagnosed and R'_t be the number of anal/rectal gonorrhoea cases reported from the respective city clinics (see Fig. 5.4). Transmission is a function of the contact rate between infectious and uninfected individuals and is assumed to depend on the relative rather than absolute number of susceptible individuals (Getz and Pickering 1983). If it is assumed that the contact rate function for AIDS is the same as that for anal/rectal gonorrhoea, R'_t reflects the changes in sexual behaviour that have occurred.

The length of time from exposure to diagnosis with AIDS is characterized by a constant δ. Infectious individuals are assumed to transmit the disease agent starting $\delta-\mu$ months after exposure until σ months before diagnosis.

In characterizing saturation, the model uses the parameter $\kappa_a = 1/N(1-\nu)$, where N is the population size and ν is the proportion of exposed individuals that will never develop the severest form of the disease and be diagnosed with AIDS.

The parameters κ_g and κ are composite terms that include scalars for the relative infectivity of gonorrhoea and AIDS. In the following analysis these parameters are free. Their values are chosen to give the best fit of the model to observations.

5. Computer code and parameter estimation

Each expected value of D_t generated by the model depends on the values of the parameters δ, μ, σ, κ_a, κ_g, and κ, and on the numbers of AIDS and anal/rectal gonorrhoea cases in the periods specified by the appropriate parameters. We have used IBM microcomputers to iterate through numerous sets of δ, μ, σ, κ_a, and κ_g values. For each set, a program named AFIT solves for the κ value that best fits the model by the least-squares criterion to the observed AIDS incidence for the months t_1 to t_2, which in the following analysis are April 1983 and March 1986 respectively. AFIT stores the set of σ, κ, κ_a, and κ_g values with the lowest sum-of-squares value for each pair of possible δ values (integers ranging from 1 to 120) and $\delta-\mu$ values (integers ranging from zero to 18) in a sequential file for each city. Thus the original code has been modified to allow disease development times of up to 120 months.

Once parameter values are chosen, additional computer programs forecast AIDS incidence and plot the model's output against observations. The model code is available from JP.

6. Sensitivity analysis

In a previous paper (Pickering *et al.* 1986), we considered unrestricted parameter sets. Our results showed that sets yielding similar fits to observations could give radically different forecasts of the epidemic. Ideally, we wish to fix all parameter values with data from independent studies. In reality, given our current knowledge of AIDS, we can only partially restrict the values of κ_a and δ. We now make these restrictions and show the model's sensitivity to ranges in parameter values.

The San Francisco City Clinic Cohort Study provides details of the proportion of HIV-seropositive men who develop AIDS as a function of time since seroconversion (Hessol *et al.* 1987). This study, which is based on a Kaplan–Meier time-to-progression analysis, estimates that 5 per cent, 10 per cent, 15 per cent, 24 per cent, 30 per cent, and 36 per cent of HIV-infected men will develop AIDS within 36 months, 48 months, 60 months, 72 months, 84 months and 88 months after seroconversion respectively. Although the 95 per cent confidence interval for the final quoted value is 26–46 per cent, only 22 per cent of the men are completely asymptomatic after an average follow-up of 76 months, having neither AIDS, AIDS-related conditions, nor generalized lymphadenopathy.

Based on this study, we set the disease's development time δ at a minimum of 3 years and use 6 years as the most likely value. Furthermore, we restrict ν between 0.22 (i.e. all but the asymptomatic individuals will progress to AIDS) and 0.64 (i.e. the maximum estimate of 36 per cent will not increase).

We set the population size N in San Francisco at risk of AIDS at the start of the epidemic at between 42 000 and 70 000. These values bound estimates based on two surveys, and our best estimate is that $N = 60\ 000$ (Lemp 1987).

Figure 5.5 projects the epidemic in San Francisco with κ_a restricted, on the basis of the above ranges for N and ν, between 0.000018 and 0.000066. For this graph, AIDS cases are assumed to develop in 6 years and to be continually infectious throughout this period. The parameters κ_g and κ are chosen so as to best fit the model to the observations from April 1983 to March 1986. The worst scenario (top line) has the largest population size ($N = 70\ 000$) and 78 per cent of exposed individuals progressing to AIDS. The best scenario (bottom line) has the smallest population size ($N = 42\ 000$) and only 36 per cent of exposed individuals progressing to AIDS. The two intermediate lines consider κ_a values based on $N = 60\ 000$. In the one with $\kappa_a = 0.000036$, 46 per cent of exposed individuals progress to AIDS (i.e. the upper bound of the 95 per cent confidence interval of the Kaplan–Meier-based estimate), and in the one with $\kappa_a = 0.000046$, 36 per cent progress to AIDS. Clearly, given the spread of the projections, N and ν are important parameters that need to be restricted further.

Figure 5.6 shows the effect of development time on the epidemic for the

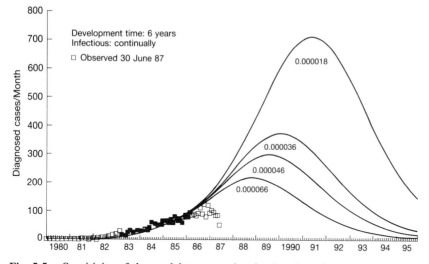

Fig. 5.5. Sensitivity of the model to saturation for San Francisco. San Francisco's AIDS incidence is modelled using anal/rectal gonorrhoea cases from San Francisco. The squares represent observed monthly AIDS incidence as reported by 30 June 1987 and underestimate the true values, particularly for the most recent months. The solid squares were fitted to estimate the values of the free parameters. The residual sums of squares (SS) compare a line's fit with the solid and not the open squares. Each line shows the output of the model for a set of parameters. The four lines illustrate the sensitivity of the model to the saturation parameter κ_a in the range 0.000018–0.000066. For this figure, we set $\delta = 72$, $\delta - \mu = 0$ and $\sigma = 0$. We let κ_g and κ be free, and estimated their values using AFIT. For the top line, $\delta = 72$, $\delta - \mu = 0$, $\sigma = 0$, $\kappa = 0.054$, $\kappa_a = 0.000018$, $\kappa_g = 0.00000$, and SS = 4982. For the second line, $\delta = 72$, $\delta - \mu = 0$, $\sigma = 0$, $\kappa = 0.055$, $\kappa_a = 0.000036$, $\kappa_g = 0.00000$, and SS = 4694. For the third line, $\delta = 72$, $\delta - \mu = 0$, $\sigma = 0$, $\kappa = 0.056$, $\kappa_a = 0.000046$, $\kappa_g = 0.00000$, and SS = 4534. Finally, for the bottom line, $\delta = 72$; $\delta - \mu = 0$, $\sigma = 0$, $\kappa = 0.058$, $\kappa_a = 0.000066$, $\kappa_g = 0.00000$, and SS = 4214.

intermediate κ_a value of 0.000036. The graph is constructed in a similar manner to Fig. 5.5 but has δ values of 36, 48, 60, or 72 months. The data after March 1986 are not used in fitting the two free parameters, and because they exceed the lower line tend to confirm that development time exceeds 3 years.

Figure 5.7 shows the effect on the epidemic's course of the length of time individuals are infectious during a development time of 72 months. As for Fig. 5.6, $\kappa_a = 0.000036$. Individuals who are infectious are assumed to start transmitting the agent immediately after exposure to it (i.e. $\delta = \mu$) and then be infectious for 7, 24, 48, or 72 months. An infectious period of 7 months (i.e. $\sigma = 65$) is presented because this gives the best fit to the solid squares for any value of σ. However, because the data after March 1986 already exceed the lower line, we tend to exclude this possibility.

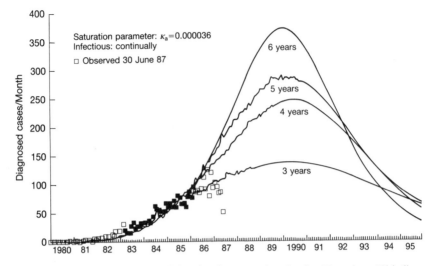

Fig. 5.6. Sensitivity of the model to development time for San Francisco. This figure uses the same representation as Fig. 5.5. The lines show the sensitivity of the model to the development time parameter δ in the range 3–6 years. For this figure we set $\kappa_a = 0.000036$, $\delta - \mu = 0$, and $\sigma = 0$, and we let κ_g and κ be free. For the top line, $\delta = 72$, $\delta - \mu = 0$, $\sigma = 0$, $\kappa = 0.055$, $\kappa_a = 0.000036$, $\kappa_g = 0.00000$ and SS = 4694. For the second line, $\delta = 60$, $\delta - \mu = 0$, $\sigma = 0$, $\kappa = 0.044$, $\kappa_a = 0.000036$, $\kappa_g = 0.00049$, and SS = 4516. For the third line, $\delta = 48$, $\delta - \mu = 0$, $\sigma = 0$, $\kappa = 0.045$, $\kappa_a = 0.000036$, $\kappa_g = 0.00050$, and SS = 4316. Finally, for the bottom line, $\delta = 36$, $\delta - \mu = 0$, $\sigma = 0$, $\kappa = 0.040$, $\kappa_a = 0.000036$, $\kappa_g = 0.00096$, and SS = 2658.

Because we are unaware of studies using random samples to determine the size of the populations at risk in New York and Los Angeles, we estimate N for these cities using the number of AIDS cases that they report relative to San Francisco. New York has approximately 3.2 times as many cases as San Francisco, and Los Angeles has approximately the same number as San Francisco. Hence, we assume that N for New York is no greater than four times the San Francisco value, and that N for Los Angeles is no greater than twice the San Francisco value. Assuming that the minimum for New York is no less than three times the minimum for San Francisco, we let N for New York range from 126 000 to 280 000. Assuming that the minimum for Los Angeles may equal the minimum for San Francisco, we let N for Los Angeles range from 42 000 to 140 000. With these ranges of N and with ν ranging from 0.22 to 0.64, we restrict κ_a to between 0.000005 and 0.000022 for New York and to between 0.000009 and 0.000066 for Los Angeles.

Figures 5.8 and 5.9 consider these κ_a ranges for New York and Los Angeles

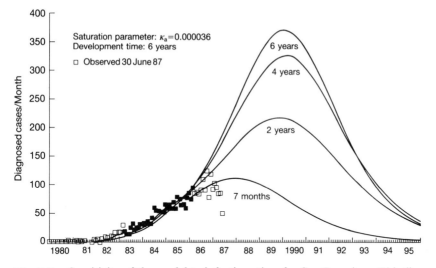

Fig. 5.7. Sensitivity of the model to infectious time for San Francisco. This figure uses the same representation as Fig. 5.5. The lines show the sensitivity of the model to the length of the infectious period $\mu - \sigma$ in the range 7 months to 6 years. For this figure, we set $\kappa_a = 0.000036$, $\delta = 72$, and $\delta - \mu = 0$, and we let κ_g and κ be free. For the top line, $\delta = 72$, $\delta - \mu = 0$, $\sigma = 0$, $\kappa = 0.055$, $\kappa_a = 0.000036$, $\kappa_g = 0.00000$, and SS = 4694. For the second line, $\delta = 72$, $\delta - \mu = 0$, $\sigma = 24$, $\kappa = 0.056$, $\kappa_a = 0.000036$, $\kappa_g = 0.00000$, and SS = 4498. For the third line, $\delta = 72$, $\delta - \mu = 0$, $\sigma = 48$, $\kappa = 0.069$, $\kappa_a = 0.000036$, $\kappa_g = 0.00000$, and SS = 2852. Finally, for the bottom line, $\delta = 72$, $\delta - \mu = 0$, $\sigma = 65$, $\kappa = 0.168$, $\kappa_a = 0.000036$, $\kappa_g = 0.00030$, and SS = 1958.

respectively. As in Fig. 5.5, they are based on the assumptions that AIDS takes 6 years to develop and that infectious individuals are contagious for 6 years. The middle lines in these figures show κ_a values calculated for the assumptions that 46 per cent of exposed individuals progress to AIDS and that $N = 200\ 000$ and $N = 90\ 000$ for New York and Los Angeles respectively. As shown in Figs 5.6 and 5.7 for San Francisco, if we consider shorter development times or shorter infectious periods, the forecasts for New York and Los Angeles in Figs 5.8 and 5.9 are too high.

7. Conclusions

If models rely solely on statistical fits to data and do not encapsulate the forces behind the phenomena that they are modelling, they are likely to be limited in their ability to forecast events. While the AIDS outbreak may have initially increased exponentially, it cannot continue to do so indefinitely because host population sizes are finite. Models based on exponential functions might predict disease incidence successfully during the onsets of epidemics. However, without the ability to predict when incidence will level

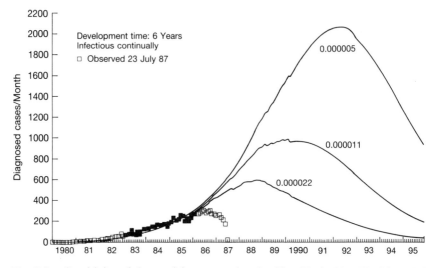

Fig. 5.8. Sensitivity of the model to saturation for New York. New York's AIDS incidence is modelled using anal/rectal gonorrhoea cases from New York. This figure uses the same representation as Fig. 5.5, with squares showing cases reported by 23 July 1987. The lines show the sensitivity of the model to the saturation parameter κ_a in the range 0.000005–0.000022. For this figure, we set $\delta = 72$, $\delta - \mu = 0$, and $\sigma = 0$, and we let κ_g and κ be free. For the top line, $\delta = 72$, $\delta - \mu = 0$, $\sigma = 0$, $\kappa = 0.044$, $\kappa_a = 0.000005$, $\kappa_g = 0.00023$, and SS = 42 350. For the second line, $\delta = 72$, $\delta - \mu = 0$, $\sigma = 0$, $\kappa = 0.044$, $\kappa_a = 0.000011$, $\kappa_g = 0.00027$, and SS = 39 206. Finally, for the bottom line, $\delta = 72$, $\delta - \mu = 0$, $\sigma = 0$, $\kappa = 0.044$, $\kappa_a = 0.000022$, $\kappa_g = 0.00036$, and SS = 33 429.

off, such models must eventually fail. If a model is to forecast disease incidence over any extended period of time, it must be based on the underlying epidemiology rather than on mathematical functions that fit existing data.

The model that we have developed attempts to encapsulate the epidemiology of AIDS incidence. However, it is not a finished product and could be improved in several ways. Its assumption that individuals develop AIDS in a fixed amount of time after exposure is a first approximation. Individuals exhibit considerable variance in the time it takes them to progress to AIDS (Goedert *et al.* 1986; Hessol *et al.* 1987), and a more sophisticated function for development time could clearly be added to the model. Another improvement concerns the way in which changes in sexual contact are indexed. Obviously, we would feel more confidence in the model if our relatively simplistic gonorrhoea model were replaced with a more realistic one (e.g. those of Hethcote and Yorke 1984, or Kramer 1980). While we work towards such improvements, the model still serves a useful purpose. It focuses attention on our lack of knowledge about specific parameters that are fundamental to understanding the epidemic and its future course.

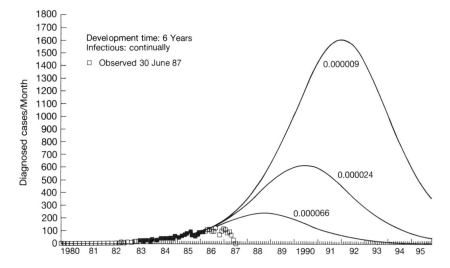

Fig. 5.9. Sensitivity of the model to saturation for Los Angeles. Los Angeles' AIDS incidence is modelled using anal/rectal gonorrhoea cases from San Francisco. This figure uses the same representation as Fig. 5.5, with squares showing cases reported by 30 June 1987. The lines show the sensitivity of the model to the saturation parameter κ_a in the range 0.000009–0.000066. For this figure we set $\delta = 72$, $\delta - \mu = 0$, and $\sigma = 0$, and we let κ_g and κ be free. For the top line, $\delta = 72$, $\delta - \mu = 0$, $\sigma = 0$, $\kappa = 0.060$, $\kappa_a = 0.000009$, $\kappa_g = 0.00000$, and SS = 4656. For the second line, $\delta = 72$, $\delta - \mu = 0$, $\sigma = 0$, $\kappa = 0.061$, $\kappa_a = 0.000024$, $\kappa_g = 0.00000$, and SS = 4468. Finally, for the bottom line, $\delta = 72$, $\delta - \mu = 0$, $\sigma = 0$, $\kappa = 0.065$, $\kappa_a = 0.000066$, $\kappa_g = 0.00000$, and SS = 3949.

As other studies involving epidemic models have concluded, more population studies of AIDS are needed (May and Anderson 1987; Anderson, Medley, Blythe, and Johnson 1987). There is a critical need for (1) randomized surveys to give better estimates of the size of the populations at risk, (2) quantification of the infectivity of exposed individuals over time, (3) better understanding of the impact of behavioural changes on transmission and disease progression, and (4) continued elucidation of the distribution of development times and the proportion of infections that develop AIDS.

Given the model's assumptions, our analysis suggests that the AIDS epidemic should peak in the three cities before 1993. Because of the model's sensitivity to the parameter values considered, it is difficult to predict the magnitude of the peaks. Nevertheless, until AIDS development times generally exceed 6 years, we suggest that Figs. 5.5, 5.8, and 5.9 can be used to provide upper bounds on the future number of cases in the cities.

References

Anderson, R.M., Medley, G.F., Blythe, S.P., and Johnson, A.M. (1987). Is it possible to predict the minimum size of the acquired immunodeficiency syndrome (AIDS) epidemic in the United Kingdom? *Lancet* **i**, 1073–5.

Drucker, E. (1987). Personal communication. Albert Einstein College of Medicine, New York.

Fox, R., Ostrow, D. Valdisseri, R., Van Raden, M., Visscher, B., and Polk, B.F. (1987). Changes in sexual activities among participants in the Multicenter AIDS Cohort Study. *3rd International Conference on Acquired Immunodeficiency Syndrome (AIDS), Washington, DC, 1–5 June*, p. 213. Bio-Data Publishers, Washington DC 1987.

Getz, W.M. and Pickering J. (1983). Epidemic models: thresholds and population regulation. *American Naturalist* **121**, 892–8.

Goedert, J.J., Biggar, R.J., Weiss, S.H., Eyster, M.E., Melbye, M., Wilson, S., Ginzburg, H.M., Grossman, R.J., DiGiola, R.A., Sanchez, W.C., Giron, J.A., Ebbeson, P., Gallo, R.C., and Blattner, W.A. (1986). Three year incidence of AIDS in five cohorts of HTLV-III-infected risk group member. *Science* **231**, 992–5.

Golubjatnikov, R., Pfister, J., and Tillotson, T. (1983). Homosexual promiscuity and the fear of AIDS. *Lancet* **ii**, 681.

Grant, R.M., Wiley, J.A., and Winkelstein, W. (1987). Infectivity of the human immunodeficiency virus: estimates from a prospective study of homosexual men. *Journal of Infectious Diseases* **156**, 189–93.

Hessol, N.A., Rutherford, G.W., O'Malley, P.M., Doll, L.S., Darrow, W.W., Jaffe, H.W., Lifson, A.R., Engelman, J.G., Maus, R., Werdegar, D., and Curran, J.W. (1987). The natural history of human immunodeficiency virus infection in a cohort of homosexual and bisexual men: a 7-year prospective study. *3rd International Conference on Acquired Immunodeficiency Syndrome (AIDS), Washington DC, 1–5 June*, p. 1. Bio-Data Publishers, Washington DC 1987.

Hethcote, H.W., and Yorke, J.A. (1984). Gonorrhea transmission dynamics and control. *Lecture Notes in Biomathematics* **56**.

Judson, F.N. (1983). Fear of AIDS and gonorrhea rates in homosexual men. *Lancet* **ii**, 159–60.

Kramer, M.A. (1980). Cost-effectiveness of screening, contact tracing, and vaccination as alternative gonorrhoea control strategies using a computer simulation model. Ph.D Thesis, Ohio State University, Columbus, Ohio 343 pp.

Lemp, G. (1987). Personal communication. City and County of San Francisco Department of Public Health.

McKusick, L., Horstman, W., and Coates, T. (1985). AIDS and sexual behaviour reported by gay men in San Francisco. *American Journal of Public Health* **75**, 493–6.

Martin, J. (1987). The impact of AIDS on gay male sexual behaviour patterns in New York City. *American Journal of Public Health* **77**, 578–81.

May, R.M. and Anderson, R.M. (1987). Transmission dynamics of HIV infection. *Nature, London* **326**, 137–42.

Morgan, W.M. (1987). Personal communication. CDC, Atlanta, Georgia.

Moss, A.R., Bacchetti, P., Osmond, D., Dritz, S., Abrams, D., Conant, M., Volberding, P., and Ziegler, J. (1985). Incidence of the acquired immunodeficiency syndrome in San Francisco, 1980–1983. *Journal of Infectious Diseases* **152**, 152–61.

Pickering, J., Wiley, J.A., Padian, N.S., Lieb, L.E., Echenberg, D.F., and Walker, J. (1986). Modelling the incidence of acquired immunodeficiency syndrome (AIDS) in San Francisco, Los Angeles, and New York. *Mathematical Modelling* **7**, 661–88.

Pickett, S.B., Bart, M., Bye, L.L., and Amory, J. (1985). Self-reported behavioral change among gay and bisexual men—San Francisco. *Morbidity and Mortality Weekly Report* **34** (40), 613–5.

Schultz, S., Friedman S., Kristal, A., and Sencer, D.J. (1984). Declining rates of rectal and pharangeal gonorrhea among males—New York City. *Morbidity and Mortality Weekly Report* **33** (21), 295–7.

Staff Report (1983). Update: acquired immunodeficiency syndrome (AIDS)—United States. *Morbidity and Mortality Weekly Report* **32** (30), 389–91.

Staff Report (1985). Revision of the case definition of acquired immunodeficiency syndrome for national reporting—United States. *Morbidity and Mortality Weekly Report* **34** (25) 373–5.

Werdegar, D., O'Malley, P., Bodecker, T., Hessol, N., and Echenberg, D. (1987). Self-reported changes in sexual behaviors among homosexual and bisexual men from the San Francisco City Clinic Cohort. *Morbidity and Mortality Weekly Report* **36** (12), 187–9.

6

Reconstruction and prediction of spread of HIV infection in populations of homosexual men

J.A.M. van Druten, Th. de Boo, A.G.M. Reintjes, J.C. Jager, S.H. Heisterkamp, R.A. Coutinho, J.M. Bos, and E.J. Ruitenberg

1. Introduction

Using data from The Netherlands and the San Francisco Center for Disease Control (CDC) cohort study attempts are made to construct dynamic models for the spread of the HIV infection in populations of homosexual men. Three distinct phases of the epidemic are considered: the spread of the infection before cases with AIDS are detected, the period in which the first cases are seen, and the period thereafter in which awareness of AIDS may lead to changes in sexual lifestyle. Figure 6.1 shows a diagrammatic presentation of these phases in a cohort of N persons (e.g. $N = 10\ 000$), where N' is the maximum number at risk in the cohort ($N - N'$ persons do not contribute to the epidemic). Point A can be situated in phase 1 (all N' persons are already at risk before cases with AIDS become visible) or in phase 2 (not all are yet at risk).

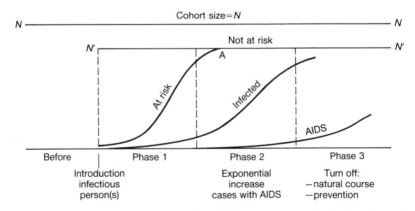

Fig. 6.1. A diagrammatic representation of the spread of HIV infection in a cohort of homosexual men.

A model for phase 1 of the epidemic is formulated in which the size of the population at risk is a dynamic variable rather than some specified constant. Two issues are addressed: (a) the reconstruction of the course of the number infected and (b) the increase in the size of the community at risk (Section 4). Phase 2 is characterized by an exponential increase in the number of cases with AIDS. Here the main question concerns the number already infected with HIV (Section 5). With regard to phase 3 of the epidemic an attempt is made to predict the long-term prevalence of the infection in high risk homosexual communities (Section 6).

Table 6.1 presents the cumulative number of cases with AIDS in The Netherlands (Geneeskundige Hoofdinspectie) and the San Francisco (SF) CDC cohort (Curran, Meade Morgan, Hardy, Jaffe, Darrow, and Dowdle 1985). The cases with AIDS in The Netherlands are predominantly homosexuals located in Amsterdam (90 per cent). The data for the SF cohort come from a study of hepatitis B in 6 875 homosexual and bisexual men performed in 1978. The reason for the inclusion of these data in the analysis of the Dutch data is threefold: firstly the size of the SF cohort is known and the growth rate of the epidemic in phase 2 is the same as that observed in The Netherlands (Section 2), secondly we can test and validate mathematical models using the SF data (Section 3), and thirdly we can learn from these data simply because there is a time delay between the onset of the two epidemics.

In fact two kinds of main data are available from San Francisco for mathematical analysis—the data briefly summarized in Table 6.1 and data from the city of San Francisco as a whole. The latter have been subjected to mathematical modelling by Bailey and Estreicher (1986). The only data on homosexuals *per se* at risk comes from the SF CDC cohort study (San Francisco City Clinic). The study provides longitudinal data—serological and cases with AIDS—from the longest time window currently available. Further information with respect to this study can be found in Jaffe *et al.* (1985), Echenberg, Rutherford, O'Malley, and Bodecker (1985), and Enstrom (1986). A preliminary mathematical analysis of the summarized data (Table

Table 6.1. AIDS epidemic in The Netherlands and in the San Francisco CDC cohort.

Year	1978	1979	1980	1981	1982	1983	1984	1985	1986
The Netherlands†									
AIDS cumulative	0	0	0	0	3	18	48	106	218
SF CDC cohort ($n = 6875$)‡									
AIDS cumulative	0	0	2	14	41	84	166		
Number seropositive	275	825	1650	2406	3162	3919	4675		

†Source: Geneeskundige Hoofdinspectie.
‡Source: Curran *et al.* 1985.

6.1) has been given by van Druten, de Boo, Jager, Heisterkamp, Coutinho, and Ruitenberg (1986). Mathematical derivations are presented in the Appendix.

2. Initial growth rate of the AIDS epidemic in The Netherlands

To make a comparison between the initial growth rates of the epidemic in The Netherlands and the SF cohort, a logarithmic transformation was applied to the cumulative number of cases with AIDS†. Exponential growth rates then appear as straight lines (Fig. 6.2). If the few cases reported in the first year of appearance (two cases in the SF data and three in the Dutch data) are discarded, the slopes of the lines, i.e. the growth rates of the epidemics, are the same in the initial stage of phase 2. The slope value $b = 0.89$ corresponds to a doubling time of 9 months. The size of the SF cohort and the shift in the regression lines of both epidemics are known. Therefore an attempt was made to estimate the size of the homosexual community initially at risk in The Netherlands. Since a difference between the sizes of the communities at risk influences the shift in the two regression lines, a distinction was made between the observed shift Δ (Fig. 6.2, $\Delta = 1.75$) and the (standardized) delay time d, i.e. the delay time between epidemics in the case where communities at risk would have been of equal size. For notational convenience, let n be the

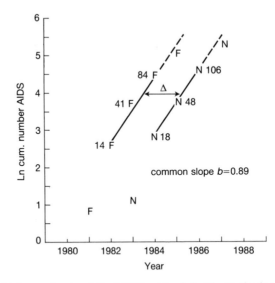

Fig. 6.2.   Initial growth rate of the AIDS epidemic in The Netherlands and in the SF CDC cohort.

† In this paper 'logarithmic' refers to the natural logarithm.

Table 6.2. Delay time *d* and size *n* of the homosexual community initially at risk in The Netherlands: comparison with the San Francisco CDC cohort study ($n_0 = 6875$).

Delay time *d* (years)	Relative size n/n_0	Size *n*
2	1.3	9 000
3	3.0	20 000
4	7.4	50 000

Application of equation (6.1) with $\Delta = 1.75$ and $b = 0.89$.

size of a study population at risk in phase 2 of the epidemic (homosexuals initially at risk in The Netherlands) and n_0 be the size of a reference population (the SF study cohort). Then the following relationship can be derived:

$$d = \Delta + \frac{\ln(n/n_0)}{b}, \tag{6.1}$$

where *b* is the initial growth rate of both epidemics (common slope). If $n = n_0$, then $d = \Delta$. If $n > n_0$, then the delay time *d* is larger than the observed shift Δ. If there is no delay in the onset of the two epidemics, $d = 0$ and then a shift Δ in the regression lines may be observed simply because the sizes of the communities at risk are different. It should be emphasized that equation (6.1) refers to phase 2 of the epidemic and that the number of cases with AIDS is considered to be proportional to the size of the population at risk. The theoretical relationship between the delay time *d* and the size *n* of the homosexual community initially at risk in The Netherlands was calculated using equation (6.1) and the values $n_0 = 6\ 875$, $b = 0.89$, and $\Delta = 1.75$, and is presented in Table 6.2. Given the delay time *d*, we can assess *n*; given the size *n*, we can estimate *d*. We cannot estimate both *d* and *n* simultaneously without further information.

The apparent countrywise delay time between the AIDS epidemic in the USA and the FRG is 3 years (L'age-Stehr 1985). If the difference between the population sizes is taken into account according to equation (6.1), the standardized delay time *d* would be approximately 2 years. If we assume a standardized delay *d* of 2–3 years between the AIDS epidemic in the SF study cohort and The Netherlands (mainly homosexuals located in Amsterdam), it is estimated that between 9000 and 20 000 homosexuals were initially at risk in The Netherlands.

3. A basic cohort model

A tentative model is now formulated to examine the simultaneous course of the number infected and the cumulative number of cases with AIDS in a cohort of homosexual men in phases 1 and 2 of the epidemic. The size n of the cohort at risk is provisionally assumed to be constant. Before the model was applied to the Dutch data, its performance and predictive behaviour were examined using the SF data (van Druten *et al.* 1986). The model is a three-parameter model with parameters β, γ, and p_a, where β is a transmission coefficient which depends on the sexual contact rate and the method of contact, e.g. unprotected anal intercourse, p_a is the probability of acquiring full-blown AIDS after infection, and $1/\gamma$ is the average duration of the infected period.

In the model the incubation period is assumed to be equal to the infected period.† A compartmental presentation is shown in Fig. 6.3. The model is an adaptation of a model proposed by Kermack and McKendrick (1927), which was discussed and extended by Bailey (1975) and Bailey and Estreicher (1986) to study the AIDS epidemic. In phase 1 and the early stage of phase 2 of the epidemic, the compartments below the broken line contain relatively small numbers of persons. The rate at which persons acquire the HIV infection is determined by the number of persons in the compartments denoted by 'susceptibles' and 'infected' according to the mass action law of epidemiology ($dy/dt = \beta xy$). The population dynamics of various infectious diseases, i.e. based on this law, are presented by Anderson (1982).

By applying the model to the SF data (Table 6.1), two basic equations can

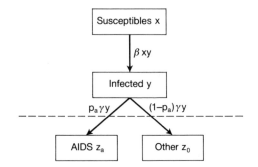

Fig. 6.3. A three-parameter cohort model. The rate at which susceptibles acquire the infection is determined by the mass action law of epidemiology, p_a is the probability of acquiring full-blown AIDS, and $1/\gamma$ is the average duration of the infected/incubation period.

† Throughout the paper the infectious period is set equal to the infected period. In Section 6 a distinction is made between the duration of the infected (infectious) periods of those who do and those who do not develop full-blown AIDS.

be used to estimate the parameters and examine the fit. The model approximately predicts an exponential increase in the cumulative number of cases with AIDS in the early stage of phase 2. Figure 6.2 and numerous papers show that this pattern is generally observed in various European countries and the USA (Anderson, Medley, May, and Johnson 1986; Downs *et al.* 1988; Gonzalez and Koch 1986; Heisterkamp *et al.* 1988; Pickering, Wiley, Padian, Lieb, Echenberg, and Walker 1986; McEvoy and Tillett 1985). This provides us with a first equation linking the parameters β and γ to the growth rate b of the epidemic (SF data, $n = 6\ 875$):

$$b = n\beta - \gamma. \tag{6.2}$$

The expression $n\beta$ can be interpreted as the annual effective contact rate, i.e. the average number of new infected persons generated by one infected person in a period of 1 year in a completely susceptible population. As shown in Fig. 6.2 the initial growth rates of the AIDS epidemics in the SF cohort and The Netherlands are the same. This indicates that the initial number of effective person contacts per person per year that results in transmission of HIV was approximately the same in both homosexual communities (assuming no difference in the distributions of the incubation periods). Table 6.3 shows that the annual effective contact rate c may have values between 0.8 and 1.7. If the average incubation period is about 5 years, c would have a value near unity. This value is of the same magnitude as the estimate for the total homosexual community in San Francisco, where the effective contact rate is 0.091 per month (Bailey and Estreicher 1986). This would imply that on average there is one potential effective contact per person per year, i.e. a contact (probably consisting of multiple sexual contacts) that will produce a new infected person if one is infected (infectious) and the other is susceptible. This is also an indication that the probability of transmission of HIV per sexual contact is low.

The model also predicts a linear relationship between ln (susceptibles) and the cumulative number of cases with AIDS:

Table 6.3. Annual effective contact rate as a function of the initial doubling time of the epidemic† and the average duration of the infected period.

Initial slope	Initial doubling time	Annual effective contact rate		
		3 years‡	5 years‡	10 years‡
0.693	1 year	1.0	0.9	0.8
0.89	~ 9 months	1.2	1.1	1.0
1.386	6 months	1.7	1.6	1.5

†SF CDC study cohort and The Netherlands: slope, 0.89; initial doubling time, about 9 months.
‡Infected period.

$$\ln x = \ln x_0 - \frac{R}{np_a} z_a, \tag{6.3}$$

where $n = 6\,875$ (SF data), x is the number of susceptibles (seronegatives), z_a is the cumulative number with AIDS, p_a is the probability of acquiring AIDS after infection, and R is the basic reproduction rate.† This leads to a second graphical examination for the fit of the model and a second equation which can be used for the estimation of the parameters. Figure 6.4 shows the relationship between $\ln x$ and z_a for the SF data presented in Table 6.1. The bivariate data points $(z_a, \ln x)$ for the years 1981, 1982, and 1983 show a linear relationship. If the model is appropriate for the study of the course of the epidemic in this period, the results would incidate that no substantial changes in sexual lifestyle had occurred before 1983. From (6.3) it immediately follows that

$$b' = -\frac{R}{np_a}. \tag{6.4}$$

By combining equations (6.2) and (6.4) and using the slope values $b = 0.89$ and $b' = -0.0058$ (Figs 6.2 and 6.4), we can obtain preliminary estimates of

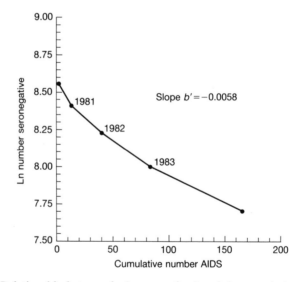

Fig. 6.4. Relationship between ln (seronegatives) and the cumulative number with AIDS obtained using data from the SF cohort.

† The basic reproduction rate of the infection is a key parameter in infectious disease epidemiology and can be defined as the average number of new infected persons generated by one primary case during his infected (infectious) period in a completely susceptible population, i.e. $R = c/\gamma$.

the average duration of the incubation period $1/\gamma$ and the basic reproduction rate R. Given values for the probability of acquiring full-blown AIDS after infection, we obtain $R = 4$ for $p_a = 0.10$ and $R = 8$ for $p_a = 0.20$. From (6.2) and the definition of the basic reproduction rate it follows that $R = 1 + b/\gamma$. The values $R = 4$ and $R = 8$ correspond to $1/\gamma = 3.4$ years and $1/\gamma = 7.9$ years respectively. Mathematical analysis of the AIDS epidemic in the total homosexual community of San Francisco (100 000 men) shows that the average incubation period is around 5 years (Bailey and Estreicher 1986). The tentative estimates of the incubation period (3.4 years and 7.9 years respectively) are roughly in agreement with this figure. By varying the slope b the range of possible values of R was studied further. The results are shown graphically in Fig. 6.5.

Building a model is one part of the problem. The determination of its range of applicability is another, often more difficult, task. For instance the question arises as to whether the model can predict the course of the epidemic in the SF cohort. On the basis of the limited data for 1978 (a retrospectively estimated 275 seropositive men and no reported cases with AIDS (Table 6.1)) and parameter estimates ($c = 1$ year^{-1}, $p_a = 0.10$, and $1/\gamma$ values of 3, 5, and 10 years), simulation studies were performed to predict the simultaneous course of the number infected and the cumulative number of cases with

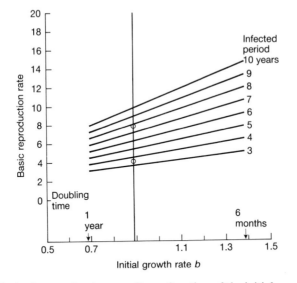

Fig. 6.5. The basic reproduction rate R as a function of the initial growth rate b of the AIDS epidemic and the average duration of the infected period $1/\gamma$. The values $R = 4$ and $R = 8$ correspond to the pairs $1/\gamma = 3.4$, $p_a = 0.10$ and $1/\gamma = 7.9$, $p_a = 0.20$ respectively (p_a is the probability of acquiring full-blown AIDS in phase 2 of the epidemic).

AIDS (van Druten *et al.* 1986). In these studies it was observed that the cases diagnosed as having AIDS were seen later than predicted by the model. There are several explanations for this discrepancy between model prediction and data. Firstly the exponential distribution tentatively used here to model the distribution of the incubation period should be replaced by another distribution. If an exponential distribution is not appropriate, a gamma (Bailey and Estreicher 1986) or a Weibull distribution (Anderson, Medley, May, and Johnson 1986) is often used. There is evidence that the distribution of incubation periods among transfusion-associated AIDS cases follows a Weibull distribution with a median of 52 months (Lui, Lawrence, Morgan, Peterman, Haverkos, and Bregman 1986). If this distribution is also applicable to sexual transmission, it may explain the delay between the time of onset of observed and predicted cases. There is also another mechanism which may explain, at least to some extent, this delay, and that is the initial increase in the size of the community at risk in phase 1 of the epidemic. This issue is explored further in the next section.

4. Spread of HIV infection before cases with AIDS are detected

After the introduction of one or more infectious persons into a cohort of, say, 10 000 homosexual men, the spread of the infection in the community occurs very slowly since the annual effective contact rate is rather low (Table 6.3). Consequently not all persons are immediately at risk of acquiring an infection; those who are at risk have sexual contacts with infected (infectious) persons. To study the spread of HIV infection and the increase in the size of the community at risk in the years before cases with AIDS are detected, a dynamic size transmission model was formulated.

At $t = 0$, it is assumed that y_0 infected/infectious persons are introduced into the cohort. The average number of sexual partners per infected person at time t is denoted by the contact parameter ρ, i.e. at $t = 0$ there are ρy_0 persons at risk of acquiring an HIV infection. The contact parameter ρ describes the number of partners per infected person at time t; it depends on the rate of change of partners and the duration of the partnership. The objective is to study the simultaneous course of the number infected $y(t)$ and the size $n(t)$ of the community at risk. At time t the size $n(t)$ consists of the number $y(t)$ already infected and the number of partners at time t who are susceptible. Note that this formation is changing with time. Following the notation shown in Fig. 6.1, the dynamics of $y(t)$ and $n(t)$ are described by the following set of differential equations:

$$x(t) + y(t) = n(t) \qquad\qquad n(t) \leqslant N' \qquad\qquad (6.5)$$

$$\frac{dy}{dt} = \beta xy \qquad\qquad \beta\{n(t)\}n(t) = c \qquad\qquad (6.6)$$

$$\frac{dn}{dt} = \rho \left\{ 1 - \frac{n(t)}{N'} \right\} \frac{dy}{dt} \qquad y(0) = y_0 \text{ and } n(0) = (\rho + 1)y_0. \quad (6.7)$$

The maximum number of persons at risk is N'; therefore we have $n(t) \leqslant N'$. The annual effective contact rate c can be expressed in terms of n and β; $c = n\beta$. It is unlikely that the sexual lifestyle of homosexuals had already changed before cases with AIDS were diagnosed; therefore c is regarded as a constant in phase 1 of the epidemic. Because n is a dynamic variable it follows that the transmission coefficient $\beta(t)$ is decreasing with time. The growth rate dn/dt of the number of persons at risk is considered to be proportional to the growth rate dy/dt of the number infected and the average number ρ of (sexual) partners per infected person at time t multiplied by $1 - n(t)/N'$, i.e. to take into account persons already at risk.

The model can be considered to be an extension of the conventional epidemic model with $dn/dt = 0$. *A priori* we might assume that a model in which the size of the community at risk is a dynamic variable, rather than some specified constant, is more realistic. To examine the difference between the two models, approximate solutions for the number infected $y(t)$ and the number $n(t)$ of persons at risk were derived. The size n of the community at risk was updated each year and within that period the mass action law was applied to determine the course of the number infected $y(t)$. The overall course of $y(t)$ was described by piecewise logistic functions. The estimates of the effective contact rate c presented in Table 6.3 were used in an attempt to reconstruct the course of the number infected in the SF study cohort. The value of the contact parameter ρ was varied over a wide range, and it was assumed that one infected (infectious) person was introduced into the cohort at $t = 0$.

Figure 6.6 shows the course of the number infected as predicted by the dynamic-size model with $\rho = 10$ and the conventional model ($dn/dt = 0$, $n = N' = 6\ 875$). Up to the diagnosis of the first two AIDS cases (in 1980) the numbers of seropositive persons estimated retrospectively were 275 (1978), 825 (1979) and 1 650 (1980) (see Table 6.1). The data do not discriminate clearly between the two models. To show that in principle the dynamic size model could explain the spread of HIV infection before AIDS cases are detected, these data points are drawn in Fig. 6.6, curve b. This curve corresponds to the parameter values $\rho = 10$, $c = 1.1\ \text{year}^{-1}$ and $1/\gamma = 5$ years. The following observation can be made regarding the pattern of the curves $y(t)$ of the constant-size and dynamic-size models. In the dynamic-size model the growth rate of the number infected $y(t)$ is clearly slower in the first few years after the start of the epidemic, and as a result the time interval required to attain a cumulative number of 1650 seropositives is clearly longer. Therefore it can be concluded that in a dynamic-size model AIDS cases are predicted later than in the constant-size model. Figure 6.6 suggests that 7 years may

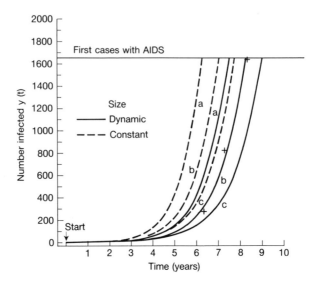

Fig. 6.6. Model reconstruction of the course of the number of persons infected in the period before cases with AIDS are detected. The constant-size model and the variable-size model (contact parameter $\rho = 10$) are compared. Curves a, b, and c are for annual effective contact rates of 1.2, 1.1, and 1.0 with incubation periods of 3 years, 5 years and 10 years respectively. The data points + correspond to 275, 825, and 1650 seropositives in the SF CDC study cohort (Table 6.1). Points are drawn for illustration on curve b of the variable-size model.

elapse after the introduction of the first infected (infectious) person(s) into the community before the first AIDS cases are seen. If this applies to The Netherlands, the first infected person may have started the epidemic in 1975 (the first cases were detected in 1982 (Table 6.1)).

The simultaneous course of the number infected $y(t)$ and the number at risk $n(t)$ in the dynamic-size model is shown in Fig. 6.7. According to the model, all persons in a high risk population of the same size as the SF study cohort are already at risk before the first cases with AIDS are detected, provided that homogeneous mixing can be assumed and that at time t the average contact parameter ρ is about 10 or more per infected person. In a study of 741 homosexual men in Amsterdam in the period October 1984–1986 the average number of sexual partners per individual over a period of 6 months before the examination was 20 men, of whom 50 per cent were anonymous (van Grien-sven, Tielman, Goudsmit, van der Noordaa, de Wolf, and Coutinho 1986).

When the value of the contact parameter ρ is very low or the size of the community at risk is very large, not everyone is at risk before the risk cases with full-blown AIDS are detected. This situation is expressed by the position of point A in Fig. 6.1. This figure also shows that not everyone in a

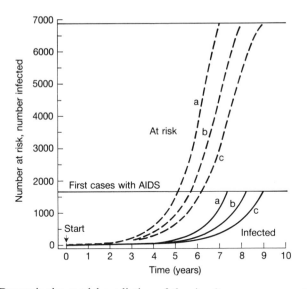

Fig. 6.7 Dynamic size model prediction of the simultaneous course of the number infected and the number at risk (contact parameter $\rho = 10$). Curves a, b, and c are as defined in Fig. 6.6.

cohort need be at risk in phase 2 of the epidemic. If the community is heterogeneous with respect to sexual lifestyle, as seems probable in the total homosexual community in San Francisco, mathematical analysis suggests that 32 per cent of the men do not contribute to the epidemic (Bailey and Estreicher 1986). This would still leave 70 000 homosexuals at risk.

6.5 Number already infected

The three-parameter model described in Section 3 was tentatively used to predict the number s^+ already infected (serologically positive individuals) from the cumulative number z_a of cases with AIDS in phase 2 of the epidemic. On the basis of this model the following theoretical relationship can be derived:

$$s^+(z_a) = n \left\{ 1 - \exp\left(- \frac{1 + b/\gamma}{np_a} z_a \right) \right\}, \tag{6.8}$$

where n is the size of the cohort at risk and the parameters b, γ, and p_a are as defined earlier. This relationship was used to predict in a cohort of 10 000 persons the course of the ratio of the number already infected to the number of cases with AIDS as a function of z_a. The results are shown in Fig. 6.8(a) for various values of the parameters.

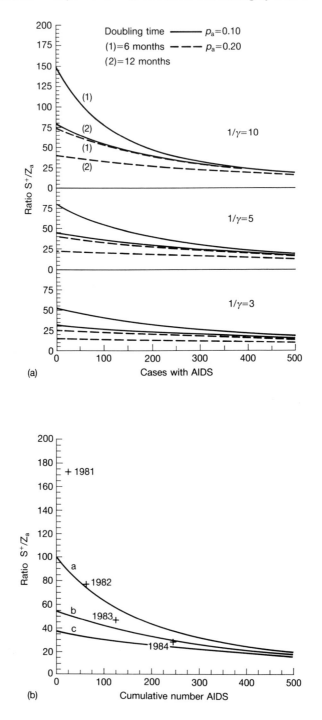

(a)

(b)

The model given by equation (6.8) predicts that in a cohort study the ratio r will decrease owing to the natural course of the epidemic. Furthermore, the ratio becomes less dependent on the initial doubling time of the epidemic, the average duration of the infected (incubation) period, and the probability of acquiring AIDS. To give an indication of how many persons are already infected relative to the cumulative number reported with AIDS, a ratio of 30–100 is often quoted. In a qualitative sense the model predictions reflect this expectation rather well.

The model predictions of the ratio r using the parameter estimate $b = 0.89$ (initial doubling time 9 months (Table 6.3)) are presented in Fig. 6.8(b). The actual ratios observed in the SF study (values derived from Table 6.1) are also shown (the cohort size was standardized to 10 000 persons at risk). If only a few cases with AIDS (z_a) are used to predict the ratio $r = s^+ / z_a$, the curves clearly underestimate the number already infected. In view of the remarks in Sections 3 and 4, this bias could be expected. For cumulative numbers of cases with AIDS, say larger than 50 per 10 000, the bandwidths of the three curves reflect the course of the ratio r as observed in the SF study. In phase 2 of the epidemic the model with $p_a = 0.10$ appears to fit the data better than the model with $p_a = 0.20$. This result is in qualitative agreement with the estimate that, until 1985, 6.4 per cent (95 per cent confidence interval, 0.8–21.4 per cent) of men who were seropositive for more than 5 years have acquired AIDS in the SF cohort (Jaffe *et al.* 1985). In the long run estimates of the probability of acquiring AIDS after infection will substantially increase. As explained, the three-parameter model can only be used in a particular phase of the epidemic to estimate, sometimes in a rather crude sense, certain epidemiological parameters. Outside this range the model is of limited value.

The curves in Fig. 6.8(b) were used to estimate the number infected in the homosexual community initially at risk in The Netherlands. Given 200 homosexuals diagnosed with AIDS and the provisional estimates of the numbers at risk (Table 6.2), we might assume that between 5000 and 15 000 homosexuals in this community were infected at the end of 1986 (Table 6.4). These estimates do not take into account the possibility that the infected individuals do not belong to the homosexual community initially at risk. The infection is probably slowly spreading to other communities, including heterosexual

---

Fig. 6.8. (a) Model predictions of the ratio of the number s^+ already infected to the cumulative number z_a of cases with AIDS in phase 2 of the epidemic (the data refer to 10 000 men at risk in a cohort study, p_a is the probability of acquiring full-blown AIDS, and $1/\gamma$ is the average duration of the infected (incubation) period in years); (b) the ratio s^+ / z_a in the SF CDC cohort study compared with model predictions with parameter values $b = 0.89$ (i.e. initial doubling time is 9 months) and $p_a = 0.10$ (the values of z_a are standardized to $n = 10\ 000$; curves a, b, and c refer to $1/\gamma$ values of 10 years, 5 years, and 3 years respectively).

Table 6.4.   Homosexual men initially at risk in The Netherlands.

Initial size of the community at risk	Model prediction of the number infected		
	3 years†	5 years†	10 years†
9 000	5000	6300	8 000
20 000	6100	8400	12 600
50 000	6800	9800	16 400

Estimates of the number infected given 200 cumulative cases of full-blown AIDS. The figures are conditionally on the size of the community at risk and the average values of the incubation period (b = 0.89, $1/\gamma$ = 3, 5 or 10 years, p_a = 0.10).
†Incubation period.

communities, in other parts of The Netherlands. Models for the dynamics of the spread of HIV infection in the heterosexual population are presented by Dietz (1986) and Knox (1986).

Even if the transmission of HIV could be completely blocked today, we might expect that some 2 000 people will develop AIDS in The Netherlands in the next decade. This is of course a minimum number; transmission is still going on. The projected minimum size of the epidemic in the USA is 50 times larger. Between 1986 and 1991 102 000 new cases are projected with a total cumulative incidence of 135 000 AIDS cases (Brookmeyer and Gail 1986).

6.6 Long-term prediction

Projections of the size of the AIDS epidemic are of major importance for future health care and prevention. It is estimated that by 1991 some 270 000 people in the USA will have AIDS or will have died from the disease. This is twice the projected minimum number. What really is uncertain, however, is how many people will become infected (Barnes 1986). If we restrict the projections to the high-risk homosexual communities, we can give tentative estimates of the long-term prevalence of HIV in these populations. Important questions to be addressed are as follows: (a) What will be the long-term prevalence without change in sexual lifestyle? (b) What will be the effect of a reduction in the annual effective contact rate?

To provide answers to the first question the three-parameter model (Section 3) was extended. A schematic diagram is presented in Fig. 6.9. Those persons who develop full-blown AIDS after infection and those who do not are classified in separate classes. The sexual lifestyle and the actual time window of sexual activity of the persons in these two classes are essential factors in the prediction of long-term prevalence. The period of sexual activity after infection of those who are going to develop AIDS is

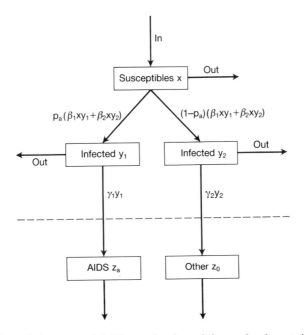

Fig. 6.9. Extended open model. Those who do and those who do not develop full-blown AIDS are classified in class 1 and class 2 respectively. The average durations of the infected periods are $1/\gamma_1$ and $1/\gamma_2$. 'In' and 'Out' refer to the time (age) window of high risk sexual activity, p_a is the probability of acquiring full-blown AIDS after infection, and β_1 and β_2 are transmission coefficients.

approximately equal to the incubation period. Of particular interest is the potential impact of those persons who do not develop full-blown AIDS after infection. Although these men may develop some other disorder, they could continually infect others over a very long period of time. The effect would be a substantial increase in the average basic reproduction rate.

We have distinguished two classes of infected persons. Therefore the average basic reproduction rate R is a weighted combination of the basic reproduction rates of persons in each of these classes:

$$R = p_a \frac{c_1}{\alpha + \gamma_1} + (1 - p_a) \frac{c_2}{\alpha + \gamma_2}, \qquad (6.9)$$

where p_a is the probability of acquiring AIDS after infection, the c_i ($i = 1,2$) are the annual effective contact rates of persons in classes 1 and 2 respectively and $1/\alpha$ is the average time window of sexual activity in the lifetime of promiscuous homosexuals. The $1/\gamma_i$ ($i = 1,2$) are the average infected periods in classes 1 and 2 respectively. The value of the parameter $1/\alpha$ was provisionally put at 40 years; for example, a person may enter the window at

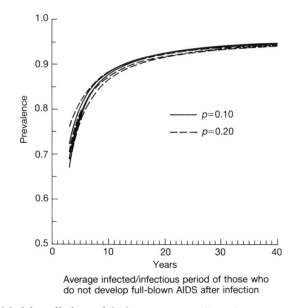

Fig. 6.10   Model predictions of the long-term prevalence for a range of values of the parameters of the extended model: $c_1 = c_2 = 1.1$ year^{-1}, $1/\alpha = 40$ years, $1/\gamma_1 = 3, 5$ or 10 years, and $p_a = 0.10$ or 0.20. Parameter $1/\gamma_2$ varies along the x axis from 3 to 40 years. See text explanation of parameters.

the age of 18 and leave at the age of 58. The long-term prevalence p refers to this time (age) window of homosexuals at risk.

In equilibrium the average net reproduction rate $R(1 - p)$ is unity†. This equation was used to estimate the long-term prevalence p as a function of the factors (parameters) presented in (6.9). The annual effective contact rate c_1 was set at 1.1 (this value corresponds to an initial doubling time of the epidemic of 9 months and an incubation period of 5 years (Table 6.3)). The effective contact rate c_2 of persons in the other class was assigned the same value (at present it is uncertain whether c_2 is larger or smaller than c_1). In order to study the potential impact of the longer time period of sexual activity of infected persons in class 2 on the prevalence of HIV, $1/\gamma_2$ was varied between 3 and 40 years. The predicted long-term prevalence is shown in Fig. 6.10. The model outcome is similar for a range of values of the parameters p_a and $1/\gamma_1$, indicating that if there is no change in sexual lifestyle HIV infection can become highly endemic in homosexual communities. The long-term prevalence could adopt a value between 70 and 90 per cent. The equilibrium of HIV infection in high risk homosexual communities

---

† The solution for the equilibrium equations is presented in the Appendix. The prevalence p includes the virtual deaths from AIDS in the defined age window.

in the UK may attain a level of 500–800 per 1000 (Knox 1986). This prediction, which takes into account heterogeneity in sexual contact rates, is somewhat lower than the figures presented here. As Anderson *et al.* (1986) have pointed out, variability in the level of sexual activity can substantially influence the predictions.

Awareness of AIDS, education, and counselling will lead to changes in sexual lifestyle, and such changes have occurred in San Francisco and other areas. According to studies by the Denver Metro Health Clinic the mean number of sexual partners for homosexual and bisexual men decreased from 5.3 to 3.2 after the respondents learned about AIDS (Riesenberg 1986)†. Those who are planning and evaluating education programmes have to predict the probable effects of such reductions. If preventive measures, e.g. reduction of sexual partners and/or changes in sexual practice, reduce the effective contact rate by a factor *f*, the question arises as to what the long-term effect will be. Figure 6.11 shows the predicted long-term prevalence of HIV infection among highly promiscuous homosexuals for a range of values of the efficacy coefficient *f*. These estimates do not take into account heterogeneity with respect to (changes in) the values of the effective contact rate. Furthermore values of fundamental parameters, e.g. p_a and c_2, are still uncertain. Consequently the following predictions are provisional. If the

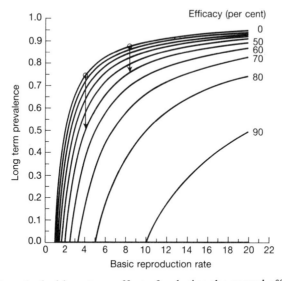

Fig. 6.11. Hypothetical long-term effect of reducing the annual effective contact rate. The arrows indicate the prediction in a situation where the efficacy of the programme is 50 per cent and the basic reproduction rate of the infection takes values of 4 and 8.

† The unit of time to which this number should refer is not reported in the paper.

basic reproduction rate R takes values between 4 and 8, the effect of reducing the effective contact rate by, for example, 50 per cent is rather limited. For values of R in this range a 90 per cent reduction in the effective contact rate should be aimed at.

The actual values of the basic reproduction rate of persons infected with HIV is clearly important in the prediction of the long-term effect of intervention programmes. Precise estimates are difficult to give. If infected persons who do not develop AIDS remain infectious for a very long period, e.g. 40 years, the average basic reproduction rate could attain a value of 20. In this situation even 90 per cent reduction of the effective contact rate might have a limited long-term effect. The infection might still be self-sustaining at a high endemic level.

Appendix 6.1.
The relationship between the shift Δ in the regression lines and the delay time d

Consider two populations π and π_0 of homosexual men at risk. The sizes are n and n_0 respectively, and π_0 is the reference population. Let $z(t)$ and $z_0(t)$ denote the cumulative number of cases with AIDS at time t in populations π and π_0 respectively. If the cumulative number of cases with AIDS in population π_0 has the value z_0 at time t_0 and if the delay time between the epidemics is d years, then we can expect nz_0/n_0 cases at time $t_0 + d$ in population π (it is assumed that the number of cases is proportional to the size of the population). This leads to the following description of $z(t)$ and $z_0(t)$:

$$z(t) = \frac{n}{n_0} z_0 \exp\{b(t - t_0 - d)\}$$

$$z_0(t) = z_0 \exp\{b(t - t_0)\},$$

where b is the common growth rate of the epidemic. The curves $z(t)$ and $z_0(t)$ appear as straight lines on a logarithmic scale. The shift Δ between these lines (see Fig. 6.2) is readily expressed in terms of the quantities n, n_0, d, and b. At time $t_0 + d$ the function $\ln\{z(t)\}$ has the value $\ln\{(nz_0/n_0)\}$. At time $t_0 + d - \Delta$ the function $\ln\{z_0(t)\}$ has the same value, i.e.

$$\ln\{z_0(t_0 + d - \Delta)\} = \ln\left(\frac{nz_0}{n_0}\right).$$

It immediately follows that

$$\ln z_0 + b(t_0 + d - \Delta - t_0) = \ln\left(\frac{nz_0}{n_0}\right),$$

and thus we have

$$d - \Delta = \frac{\ln(n/n_0)}{b}. \qquad (6.A1)$$

The difference between the shift Δ in the regression lines and the delay time d appears most pronounced in the situation where the common growth rate b of the epidemic is low.

Appendix 6.2
Basic cohort model

The dynamic model shown in Fig. 6.3 can be expressed in terms of the following differential equations ($n = x + y + z_a + z_0$):

$$\frac{dx}{dt} = -\beta xy \qquad \frac{dz_a}{dt} = p_a \gamma y$$

$$\frac{dy}{dt} = \beta xy - \gamma y \qquad \frac{dz_0}{dt} = (1 - p_a)\gamma y.$$

It is readily seen that $z_a(t) = p_a z(t)$, where $z(t) = z_a(t) + z_0(t)$. Following Bailey (1975) we have

$$\frac{dz}{dt} = \gamma y = \gamma(n - x - z).$$

By eliminating x, i.e. by using

$$\frac{dx}{dz} = -\frac{\beta}{\gamma} x \text{ and thus } x(z) = x_0 \exp\left(-\frac{\beta}{\gamma} z\right),$$

we obtain

$$\frac{dz}{dt} = \gamma \left\{ n - z - x_0 \exp\left(-\frac{\beta}{\gamma} z\right) \right\}.$$

Using a Taylor expansion and assuming $x_0 = n$, we obtain

$$\frac{dz}{dt} \approx (n\beta - \gamma)z.$$

This leads to

$$b = n\beta - \gamma, \qquad (6.A2)$$

where b is the growth rate of the cumulative number $z_a(t)$ of cases with AIDS (Fig. 6.2).

Furthermore, it immediately follows from the relationship $z_a = p_a z$ and $R = n\beta/\gamma$, where R is the basic reproduction rate, that

$$x(z_a) = x_0 \exp\left(-\frac{\beta}{\gamma}\frac{z_a}{p_a}\right),$$

and thus

$$\ln x = \ln x_0 - \frac{R}{np_a}z_a. \tag{6.A3}$$

Therefore we have

$$b' = -\frac{R}{np_a}, \tag{6.A4}$$

where b' is the value of the slope of the regression line presented in Fig. 6.4.

In order to estimate the number already infected from the cumulative number of cases with AIDS (equation (6.8) in the main text) the two relationships

$$x(z_a) = n \exp\left(-\frac{\beta}{\gamma}\frac{z_a}{p_a}\right)$$

and

$$b = n\beta - \gamma$$

were combined to give

$$x(z_a) = n \exp\left(-\frac{1 + b/\gamma}{np_a}z_a\right).$$

If the number already infected is denoted by $s^+ = n - x$, it immediately follows that

$$s^+(z_a) = n\left\{1 - \exp\left(-\frac{1 + b/\gamma}{np_a}z_a\right)\right\}. \tag{6.A5}$$

Given n, b, γ, and p_a we can estimate $s^+(z_a)$ and examine the ratio $s^+(z_a)/z_a$ as a function of the cumulative number of cases with AIDS (Fig. 6.8).

Appendix 6.3
Extended open model

In Section 6 we made preliminary long-term predictions of the prevalence of HIV infection in a community of high risk homosexual men. A brief account of the derivation of the relevant formulae is given below. The model shown in Fig. 6.9 has five compartments and the process is determined by six parameters. The size of the high risk homosexual community is denoted by n where $n = x + y_1 + y_2 + z_a + z_0$. In the absence of HIV infection the duration of active homosexual life is $1/\alpha$ years. The values of n, x, y_1, y_2, z_a, and z_0 refer to this age segment of the population. The number z_a of persons with AIDS in the defined age segment include those who have died from AIDS. Only the persons in class y_1 and y_2 generate new infected individuals. The infected (infectious) persons in class y_1, i.e. persons who will develop AIDS, have c_1y_1 effective person contacts per year. It is provisionally assumed that a fraction x/n of the contacts results in new infected persons. Hence y_1 infected persons produce β_1xy_1 new infected persons per unit time, where $\beta_1 = c_1/n$. The y_2 infected persons who will not develop AIDS produce β_2xy_2 new infected persons per unit time, where $\beta_2 = c_2/n$. A fraction p_a of infected persons will go on to develop AIDS after a mean incubation period of $1/\gamma_1$ years. The infected (infectious) period of those who will not develop AIDS in the period of active sexual life is $1/\gamma_2$ years. The differential equations used to study this system are:

$$\frac{dx}{dt} = \alpha n - \alpha x - \beta_1xy_1 - \beta_2xy_2 \tag{6.A6}$$

$$\frac{dy_1}{dt} = p_a(\beta_1xy_1 + \beta_2xy_2) - \gamma_1y_1 - \alpha y_1 \tag{6.A7}$$

$$\frac{dy_2}{dt} = (1 - p_a)(\beta_1xy_1 + \beta_2xy_2) - \gamma_2y_2 - \alpha y_2 \tag{6.A8}$$

$$\frac{dz_a}{dt} = \gamma_1y_1 - \alpha z_a \tag{6.A9}$$

$$\frac{dz_0}{dt} = \gamma_2y_2 - \alpha z_0. \tag{6.A10}$$

In what follows the emphasis is on the equilibrium equations and the determination of the fraction of the community infected with HIV, i.e. the equilibrium prevalence $p = 1 - x/n$. The conditions $dy_1/dt = 0$ and $dy_2/dt = 0$ are equivalent with

$$\begin{bmatrix} A & B \\ C & D \end{bmatrix} \begin{bmatrix} y_1 \\ y_2 \end{bmatrix} = \begin{bmatrix} 0 \\ 0 \end{bmatrix} \tag{6.A11}$$

where

$$A = p_a\beta_1x - \gamma_1 - \alpha \qquad B = p_a\beta_2x$$
$$C = (1 - p_a)\beta_1x \qquad D = (1 - p_a)\beta_2x - \gamma_2 - \alpha.$$

To obtain a non-zero solution for $\begin{bmatrix} y_1 \\ y_2 \end{bmatrix}$ with satisfies (6.A11) it is sufficient and necessary to have $\det \begin{bmatrix} A & B \\ C & D \end{bmatrix} = 0$. It immediately follows that

$$x = \frac{(\alpha + \gamma_1)(\alpha + \gamma_2)}{p_a\beta_1(\alpha + \gamma_2) + (1 - p_a)\beta_2(\alpha + \gamma_1)} \cdot \qquad (6.A12)$$

The basic reproduction rate R can be expressed as a weighted linear combination of the basic reproduction rates of the two types of infected individuals (see equation (6.9) in the main text):

$$R = p_a \frac{c_1}{\alpha + \gamma_1} + (1 - p_a) \frac{c_2}{\alpha + \gamma_2}. \qquad (6.A13)$$

This leads to $x/n = 1/R$ or $R(1 - p) = 1$. The latter equation has been used to determine the equilibrium prevalence of HIV infection as a function of the parameters incorporated in the model. Writing down all five equilibrium equations and solving the system gives

$$\frac{x}{n} = \frac{1}{R} \qquad (6.A14)$$

$$\frac{y_1}{n} = p_a \frac{\alpha(1 - 1/R)}{\alpha + \gamma_1} \qquad (6.A15)$$

$$\frac{y_2}{n} = (1 - p_a) \frac{\alpha(1 - 1/R)}{\alpha + \gamma_2} \qquad (6.A16)$$

$$\frac{z_a}{n} = p_a \frac{\gamma_1(1 - 1/R)}{\alpha + \gamma_1} \qquad (6.A17)$$

$$\frac{z_0}{n} = (1 - p_a) \frac{\gamma_2(1 - 1/R)}{\alpha + \gamma_2} \cdot \qquad (6.A18)$$

Equations (6.A15) and (6.A16) can be used to assess the relative contribution to the incidence of HIV of infected persons who respectively do and do not develop full-blown AIDS.

References

Anderson, R.M. (ed.) (1982). *Population dynamics of infectious diseases*. Chapman and Hall, London.

Anderson, R.M., Medley, G.F.H., May, R.M., and Johnson A., (1986). A preliminary study of the transmission dynamics of the human immunodeficiency virus (HIV), the causative agent of AIDS. *IMA Journal of Mathematics Applied in Medicine and Biology* 3, 229–63.

Bailey, N.T.J. (1975). *The mathematical theory of infectious disease*. Griffin, London.

Bailey, N.T.J. and Estreicher, J. (1987). Epidemic prediction and public health control, with special reference to influenza and AIDS. *Proceedings of the 1st World Congress of the Bernoulli Society, Tashkent, 8–14 September 1986*, Vol. 2, pp. 507–16. VNU Science Press.

Barnes, D.M. (1986). Grim projections for AIDS epidemic. *Science* 232, 1589–90.

Brookmeyer, R. and Gail, M.H. (1986). Minimum size of the acquired immuno-deficiency syndrome (AIDS) epidemic in the United States. *Lancet* **ii**, 1320-2.

Curran, J.W., Meade Morgan, W., Hardy, A.M., Jaffe, H.W. Darrow, W.W. and Dowdle, W.R. (1985). The epidemiology of AIDS: current status and future prospects. *Science* **229**, 1352-7.

Dietz, K. (1987). Epidemiological models for sexually transmitted infections. *Proceedings of the 1st World Congress of the Bernoulli Society, Tashkent, 8-14 September* 1986 VNU Science Press.

Downs, A.M., Ancelle, R.A., Jager, J.C., Heisterkamp, S.H., van Druten, J.A.M., Coutinho, R.A., Ruitenberg, E.J. and Brunet, J.B. (1988). The statistical estimation, from routine surveillance data, of past, present, and future trends in AIDS incidence in Europe. These *Proceedings*, pp. 1-16.

van Druten, J.A.M., de Boo, Th., Jager, J.C., Heisterkamp, S.H., Coutinho, R.A., and Ruitenberg, E.J. (1986). AIDS prediction and intervention. *Lancet* **i**, 852-3.

Echenberg, D., Rutherford, G., O'Malley, P., Bodecker, T. (1985). Update: acquired immunodeficiency syndrome in the San Francisco cohort study, 1978-85. *Morbidity and Mortality Weekly Report* **34**, 573-5.

Enstrom, J.E. (1986). AIDS among homosexual men in California. *Lancet* **i**, 975-6.

González, J.J. and Koch, M.G. (1986). On the role of the transients for the prognostic analysis of AIDS and the anciennity distribution of AIDS patients. *AIDS-Forschung (AIFO)* **11**, 621-30.

van Griensven, G.J.P., Tielman, R.A.P., Goudsmit, J., van der Noordaa, J., de Wolf, F., and Coutinho, R.A. (1986). Risikofaktoren en prevalentie van LAV/HTLV III antistoffen bij homosexuele mannen in Nederland. *Tijdschrift voor Sociale Gezondheidszorg* **64**, 100-7.

Heisterkamp, S.H., Jager, J.C., Downs, A.M., van Druten, J.A.M., and Ruitenberg, E.J., (1988). Statistical estimation of AIDS incidences from surveillance data and the link with modelling of trends. *These Proceedings*, pp. 17-25.

Jaffe, H.W., Darrow, W.W., Echenberg, D.F., O'Malley, P.M., Getchell, J.P., Kalyanaraman, V.S., Bijers, R.H., Brennan, D.P., Braff, E.H., Curran, J.W., and Francis, D.P. (1985). The acquired immunodeficiency syndrome in a cohort of homosexual men: a six-year follow-up study. *Annals of Internal Medicine* **103**, 210-14.

Kermack, W.O., and McKendrick, A.G. (1927). Contributions to the theory of epidemics (part 1). *Proceedings of the Royal Society of London, Series A* **115**, 700-21.

Knox, E.G. (1986). A transmission model for AIDS. *European Journal of Epidemiology* **2**, 165-77.

L'Age-Stehr, J. (1985). Epidemiologie von AIDS. *Öffentliche Gesundheitswesen* **47**, 343-8.

Lui, K.J., Lawrence, D.N., Morgan, W.M., Peterman, T.A., Haverkos, H.W., and Bregman, D.J. (1986). A model-based approach for estimating the mean incubation period of transfusion associated acquired immunodeficiency syndrome. *Proceedings of the National Academy of Sciences of the USA* **83**, 3051-5.

McEvoy, M. and Tillett, H.E. (1985). Some problems in the prediction of future numbers of cases of the acquired immunodeficiency syndrome in the UK. *Lancet* **ii**, 541-2.

Pickering, J., Wiley, J.A., Padian, N.S., Lieb, L.E., Echenberg, D.F., and Walker, J. (1986). Modelling the incidence of acquired immunodeficiency syndrome (AIDS) in San Francisco, Los Angeles, and New York. *Mathematical Modelling* **7**, 661–88.

Riesenberg, D.E. (1986). AIDS prompted behaviour changes reported. *Journal of the American Medical Association* **255**, 171–6.

Acknowledgements

This research was made possible by grant No. 28-1456 from the 'Praeventiefonds' (Netherlands Foundation).

7

The dynamics of spread of HIV infection in the heterosexual population

K. Dietz

1. Introduction

'. . . all epidemiology, concerned as it is with the variation of disease from time to time or from place to place, *must* be considered mathematically, however many variables are implicated, if it is to be considered scientifically at all. To say that a disease depends upon certain factors is not to say much, until we can also form an estimate as to how largely each factor influences the whole result. And the mathematical method of treatment is really nothing but the application of careful reasoning to the problem at issue.'

This quotation is due to Sir Ronald Ross who was awarded the Nobel Prize for his contributions to the detection of the transmission mode of malaria. However, he considered his mathematical contributions to the theory of epidemics to be his greatest achievement. In order to evaluate the effect of mosquito control on the prevalence of malaria he developed a mathematical model which identified the existence of a critical mosquito density below which malaria could not maintain itself at an endemic level. What Ross called his Mosquito Theorem implied that it is not necessary to eradicate mosquitos in order to eradicate malaria. Reduction below the critical level would be sufficient. This threshold concept was later verified empirically in India by finding neighbouring areas with and without malaria having mosquito densities respectively above and below the critical level. Ross's model is presented in Fig. 7.1. Both the human and the mosquito populations are divided into susceptibles and infectives, denoted here by minus and plus respectively. A susceptible human can only be infected by the bite of an infective mosquito. Similarly a susceptible mosquito can only become infected by biting an infective human host. Ross had already realized in 1911 that this mode of transmission is similar to the transmission of sexual diseases among heterosexuals. This idea was taken up by Martini (1928) in Hamburg who applied the model to the spread of syphilis. In a recent monograph by Hethcote and Yorke (1984) on the transmission dynamics of gonorrhoea this model was used to evaluate gonorrhoea control strategies in the USA.

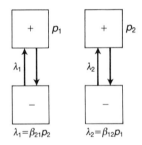

Fig. 7.1. States and transitions of the model proposed by Ross for malaria transmission which has been used by Hethcote and Yorke to describe gonorrhoea transmission in a heterosexual population. Subscripts 1 and 2 refer to the human and the vector population respectively. p_i (i = 1, 2) is the proportion infected in the ith population, and the λ_i are the infection rates which depend on the contact rates β_{12} and β_{21}.

(Unfortunately they do not give credit to the original contribution by Ross.)

In the first model used by Hethcote and Yorke the same rate of partner change was assumed for all males and females. However, they realized themselves that this rate varies considerably between individuals. In order to take this into account they divided both the male and the female population into groups with low and high rates of partner change, thus ending up with a model comprising eight compartments if the infection states are also taken into account. A similar approach has been adopted by some of the teams which have started modelling the transmission of AIDS (Table 7.1). Knox (1986) and Kiessling, Stannat, Schedel, and Deicher (1986) divide the heterosexual and homosexual population into groups according to their rates of contact (Fig. 7.2).

The drawback of this approach is the neglect of multiple contacts during a partnership. In these models it is assumed that partnerships essentially consist of one contact with which is associated a particular probability that a

Table 7.1. Preliminary list of teams involved in modelling AIDS.

Athens, GA	Pickering *et al.* 1986
Bamberg	Dörner 1986
Birmingham	Knox 1986
Geneva	Bailey and Estreicher 1987
Hanover	Kiessling *et al.* 1986
London	Anderson *et al.* 1986
Nijmegen	van Druten *et al.* 1986
Karlsborg	Koch 1985

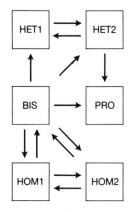

Fig. 7.2.   Subgroups of an AIDS model proposed by Kiessling *et al.* (1986): HET1, heterosexuals with a low rate of partner change; HET2, heterosexuals with a high rate of partner change; BIS, bisexuals; PRO, prostitutes; HOM1, homosexuals with a low rate of partner change; HOM2, homosexuals with a high rate of partner change.

susceptible is infected provided that the partner is infectious. As we shall see there is a large variability in the duration of partnership which has considerable implications for the dynamics of infection transmission.

Of course, the modelling of AIDS poses unique problems. There is a large body of literature on modelling measles which has been reviewed by Dietz and Schenzle (1985). In the case of measles we are dealing with an endemic disease which produces regular oscillations around a fairly stable equilibrium. Because measles is notifiable in many countries attempts at modelling have a good data base which allows alternative assumptions to be tested. In addition, the transmission dynamics are fairly homogeneous in the population if certain age-dependent factors such as higher contact rates in kindergartens and schools are taken into account. Present models allow us to assess the effects of vaccinating a certain proportion of susceptibles. On the basis of these models we can dare to predict that measles cannot be eradicated globally and we can also understand why it was possible to eradicate smallpox.

The problems with AIDS are much more difficult. We are dealing with an infection with a period of infectiousness of which neither the average duration nor the variance are known, let alone the shape of the distribution function. Because of its long average duration it will be a long time until the present epidemic reaches an equilibrium endemic state. This equilibrium state may be approached in the form of damped oscillations even if the contact rates and the infectiousness of the virus stay the same. Both parameters are likely to change. The data base which can be used to test models is of variable quality and the proportion of under-reporting is probably high. The mode of transmission involves sexual contacts and, in addition, shared use of needles, blood transfusion, and vertical transmission from mother to child. It is obvious that any modelling attempt has to be tentative and that reliable projections are impossible at present. Its main purpose is to provide a conceptual framework which helps our understanding of the transmission dynamics of the infection.

For all infectious diseases there exists a critical contact rate below which the disease cannot be maintained in an endemic state in a population. Knowledge of this critical level could help us to understand the different rates of spread in different countries and allow us to set targets to be achieved by health education programmes.

In the following we present a model which concentrates on transmission by sexual contacts. We attempt to estimate the rate of sexual contact in the heterosexual population on the basis of two surveys performed in the FRG. The other modes of transmission are ignored at this stage of model development. The paper is divided into the following sections. First, the results of questionnaire surveys of sexual behaviour in the FRG are summarized. In the next section the assumptions underlying the structure of the model are explained. A number of simulation results obtained using the model and varying some basic parameters are described in the following section. Finally, some conclusions are drawn.

2. Data on sexual behaviour

The number of sexual partners for both the homosexual and heterosexual populations has a highly skewed distribution. The variance is much larger than the mean, indicating that we are not dealing with a Poisson distribution. A survey of homosexual men by Dannecker and Reiche (1974) shows that a high rate of partner change is reported (Table 7.2). The same number of partners as is reported per year for homosexuals, i.e. 21, is reported by heterosexual males for the number of partners in a lifetime in the RALF Report (Eichner and Habermehl 1978) (Table 7.3). The number of partners of females is less than half the number of partners of males. This discrepancy can be reconciled if contacts with prostitutes are taken into account.

A more recent survey—the Sexual Education and Therapy (SEAT) Project—was published by the magazine *Stern* (Kolb 1980). Here the average numbers are considerably lower than in the RALF Report (Table 7.4). Table 7.5 reveals that about 90 per cent of both males and females state that they are in a steady partnership at present. The distribution of the duration of partnerships is given in Table 7.6. The median of this distribution is about 10 years. More than 80 per cent of both males and females state that they do not have sexual relationships outside their present partnership (Table 7.7). Table 7.8 gives the distribution of the frequency of intercourse for both males and

Table 7.2. Distribution of the number of homosexual partners during the last 12 months (Dannecker and Reiche 1974).

No. of partners	Percentage
0	0
1	7
2–5	9
6–10	16
11–20	22
21–50	20
51–100	8
100 +	7
	100 ($n = 789$)
Average number of partners	$\bar{x} = 21$
	$s = 26$

Table 7.3. Distribution of the number of sexual partners (RALF Report).

No. of sexual partners	Male (per cent)	Female (per cent)
0	<1	<1
1	11	22
2–5	22	36
6–10	27	21
11–20	14	9
21–50	11	6
51–100	7	3
100–500	4	2
500 +	<1	0
Average number of partners	$\bar{x} = 21$	$\bar{x} = 9.3$
	$s = 59$	$s = 21$

females. The average frequency is about 2.4 times per week. Of the 585 men questioned in the SEAT Project, 92.4 per cent stated that they had never had homosexual contacts (Table 7.9). However, in the survey of homosexuals by Dannecker and Reiche (1974) 16 per cent claimed that they had had at least one heterosexual contact in the preceding 12 months.

It is difficult to assess how biased these answers are. The discrepancy between the RALF Report and the SEAT Project shows the uncertainty of

Table 7.4. Number of previous sexual relationships as reported to the SEAT Project.

	Male (per cent)	Female (per cent)
None or no reply	29.8	45.7
1	7.4	11.6
2	7.9	10.2
3–5	21.3	18.9
6–10	14.6	8.9
11–20	11.4	2.7
More than 20	7.6	1.9
	100.0 ($n = 595$)	100.0 ($n = 481$)
Average number of partners	$\bar{x} = 6.2$	$\bar{x} = 2.8$
	$s = 8.2$	$s = 5.0$

Table 7.5. Data on present partnerships as reported to the SEAT Project.

	Male (per cent)	Female (per cent)
Steady partnership at present	90.9	90.4
No steady partnership at present	7.6	8.7
No sexual relationship so far	1.5	0.8
	100.0 ($n = 595$)	100.0 ($n = 481$)

Table 7.6. Data on the duration of the present partnership as reported to the SEAT Project.

	Male† (per cent)	Female† (per cent)
> 6 months	87.9	92.6
> 2 years	81.7	85.2
> 4 years	73.1	76.5
> 6 years	64.5	67.8
> 8 years	59.7	58.7
> 12 years	45.0	43.4
> 20 years	22.1	15.1

†Cumulative percentages of those who answered the question.

Table 7.7. Data on sexual relationships outside the present partnership as reported to the SEAT Project.

	Male (per cent)	Female (per cent)
Yes	14.8	11.4
No	82.9	84.6
No reply	2.4	4.0
	100.0 (*n* = 595)	100.0 (*n* = 481)

Table 7.8. Data on the average frequency of intercourse as reported to the SEAT Project.

	Male (per cent)	Female (per cent)
Never or once per year	3.7	5.2
Up to 10 times per year	1.0	0.8
Up to 3 times per month	10.1	9.6
Up to 9 times per month	2.4	4.6
Up to 2 times per month	45.2	47.4
3 times per week	21.2	18.3
4 times per week	10.8	10.2
5 times per week	6.1	0.0
Up to 9 times per week	2.2	3.5
More than 9 times per week	0.2	0.4
	100.0 (*n* = 585)	100.0 (*n* = 481)
Average (per week)	2.4	2.3
Standard deviation	1.4	1.5

Table 7.9. Data on homosexual contacts as reported to the SEAT Project†.

Very often	0.2 per cent
Frequently	0.7 per cent
Sometimes	1.7 per cent
Rarely	4.7 per cent
Never	92.4 per cent
No reply	0.3 per cent
	100.0 per cent (*n* = 585)

†Answers to the question: Did you have homosexual contacts after your 18th year of life (e.g. mutual masturbation, deep kiss, sleeping together, etc.)?

such results. However, these are the only results available for the FRG. The data provided in the Kinsey Report for the USA are probably outdated, and they have been criticized from a statistical point of view by Cochran, Mosteller and Tukey (1954). The available data are not sufficient for an epidemiological model. It is also necessary to know the average duration of the interval between partnerships and the rate at which individuals become sexually inactive in the sense that they no longer form partnerships. There is also no information about the frequency of contacts with prostitutes. In the following we make assumptions about the rates of partner change which reflect the observed values and hopefully enable us to make reasonable assumptions about the unknowns.

3. Model assumptions

The equations of the model, the definitions of the variables and the parameters, and their numerical values are given in the Appendix. The structure of the model is described below. Not all the options in the parameters were actually used to obtain the results reported here. For example, the probability of infection per contact is not necessarily symmetric in the equations but equal probabilities are assumed. Thus the computer model is far more general than the examples of simulated runs presented here suggest.

The adult male population is assumed to consist of 5 per cent homosexuals and 95 per cent heterosexuals. There is no separate class for bisexuals, i.e. it is assumed that a certain proportion of the homosexuals occasionally have contacts with females in the general population and with prostitutes (Fig. 7.3). The heterosexual male population is divided into two classes according to their rates of partner change (Table 7.10). Ninety per cent of the heterosexual males are assumed to have low rates of partner change and the remaining 10 per cent have high rates of partner change. The average duration of partnerships is 7.1 years and 1 year respectively. The average duration of the interval between two partnerships is 10 months and 4 months respectively. If it is assumed that after the termination of a partnership 2 per cent of the men decide to stay single, the present assumptions lead to an estimate of 5.6 partners per lifetime for males with low rates of partner change and 22 partners per lifetime for males with high rates of partner change. These estimates lie between those of the SEAT Project and the RALF Report. Homosexuals are assumed to have on average 10 partners per year and one heterosexual contact among single active females every 5 years. The model exists in two versions with respect to the transmission dynamics among homosexuals. The first version coincides with the classical model which assume a particular rate of single contacts with new partners per unit of time. The second version assumes a rate of formation and separation of pairs

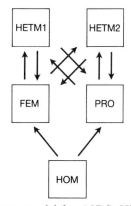

Fig. 7.3. Subgroups of present model for AIDS: HETM1 and HETM2, heterosexual males with low and high rates of partner change respectively; FEM, females
with average rate of partner change; PRO, prostitutes; HOM, homosexuals.

Table 7.10. Assumed rates of partner change.

	Males with rates of partner change	
	Low (90 per cent)	High (10 per cent)
Heterosexual		
Average duration of partnership		
(years)	7.1	1.0
Average duration of interval between		
two partnerships (months)	10	4
Probability of becoming inactive after		
the termination of a partnership		
(per cent)	2	2
Average number partners in lifetime	5.6	22.0
Homosexual		
10 homosexual partners per year		
1 heterosexual partner among single active females every 5 years		

and a contact rate within a pair. The results presented below were obtained
using the first version.

Figure 7.4 shows the dynamics of partner change in the heterosexual
population. Individuals are assumed to enter the adult population as single
actives at a certain rate. Pairs are formed which depend for males on their
category and for females on their relative abundance, and these pairs can be
terminated either by the death of one of the partners or by separation of the

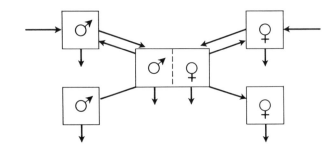

Fig. 7.4.   States and transitions of the pairing model used in this paper.

pair. At the end of a partnership the surviving partner, in the case of termination by death or each partner in the case of termination by separation decides whether he or she will re-join the active singles or will become an inactive single. The rates of contacts with female prostitutes are listed in Table 7.11. The equations in the Appendix also allow single contacts of paired males with single or paired females to be taken into account. For simplicity these are restricted to males with a high rate of partner change. Prostitutes are assumed to stay active for an average period of 8.3 years. After having been active prostitutes can either become inactive as assumed in the results given below or can join the group of single active females with an average rate of partner change. Adults have an average lifetime of 50 years. For numerical convenience the death rate is assumed to be independent of age.

Figure 7.5 shows the epidemiological assumptions made in the model. Newborns are assumed to enter the population as susceptible. This means that congenital infections are ignored. After infection an individual stays infectious for the rest of his life. The death rate in the infectious state is higher than the death rate in the susceptible state. The model does not explicitly

Table 7.11.   Assumed frequency of contact with female prostitutes.

	Males with rates of partner change	
	Low (90 per cent)	High (10 per cent)
Heterosexual		
Frequency of contact		
Single active males (per year)	0.1	5
Paired males (per year)	0	0.5
Lifetime number of contacts with		
female prostitutes	0.6	47
Homosexual		
1 contact with a female prostitute every 2 years		

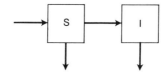

Fig. 7.5. States and transitions of the epidemiological model used in this paper.

differentiate between the various clinical manifestations of AIDS. Therefore it is only possible to calculate the incidence of new infections and the incidence of deaths due to AIDS. If there were no natural mortality the model would predict that sooner or later every infected individual would die as a result of AIDS. The probability that an infected individual dies as a result of AIDS depends on the differential death-rate due to AIDS. Data for transfusion-induced infections indicate that the average duration between infection and the end of the infectious period is about 5 years. However, some runs of the model are made using a longer infectious period.

Table 7.12 gives the assumed probabilities of infection transmission per sexual contact. Homosexual contacts, particularly those involving anal intercourse, are considered to involve a higher risk of infection than heterosexual contacts. The infection probability per contact with prostitutes is only one-third of that for contacts between heterosexuals. This may reflect the use of condoms. The initial compositions of the male and female population at the beginning of transmission, based on the assumptions made about changes of partner, are given in Tables 7.13 and 7.14. The total size of the population is assumed to be one million. Twenty-five per cent are assumed to be children and teenagers for whom the risk of sexual transmission is considered to be zero. Therefore they are not included in the model. They only appear in the denominator when rates are calculated with respect to the total population. At equilibrium about 80 per cent of the males with low rates of partner change are paired. The males with high rates of partner change are only paired at a level of 42 per cent. Because these males change partners so frequently and have a 2 per cent chance of becoming inactive after each partnership, the proportion of single inactives in this group is considerably

Table 7.12. Assumed probabilities of infection transmission per sexual contact and frequency of intercourse during a partnership.

Type of contact	
Heterosexual	1 or 2 per cent
Homosexual	10 per cent
Proportion of 'safe' contacts with female prostitutes	2/3
Frequency of intercourse (per week)	2

Table 7.13.   Composition of the male model population at the beginning of transmission.

Total size of male population	500 000
Children and teenagers	25 per cent
Adults	75 per cent
Among adult males	
Heterosexuals	95 per cent
Homosexuals	5 per cent
Among heterosexuals	
Low rates of partner change	90 per cent
High rates of partner change	10 per cent
Among males with low rates of partner change	
Single active	11.1 per cent
Paired	79.4 per cent
Single inactive	9.5 per cent
Among males with high rates of partner change	
Single active	14.6 per cent
Paired	42.3 per cent
Single inactive	43.1 per cent

Table 7.14.   Composition of the female model population at the beginning of transmission.

Total size of female population	500 000
Children and teenagers	25 per cent
Adults	75 per cent
Among adult females	
Average rates of partner change	99.9 per cent
Prostitutes (active or inactive)	0.1 per cent
Among prostitutes	
Active	16.7 per cent
Inactive	83.3 per cent
Among females with average rates of partner change	
Single active	15.8 per cent
Paired	71.9 per cent
Single inactive	12.3 per cent

higher than that for males with low rates of partner change. One female per thousand is assumed to be either an active or an inactive prostitute.

Figure 7.6 shows the states and transitions for one rate of partner change in the heterosexual population. Negative female singles can become infected by contacts with bisexuals. Negative single males can become infected by contacts with prostitutes. If a susceptible male and female form a pair then they

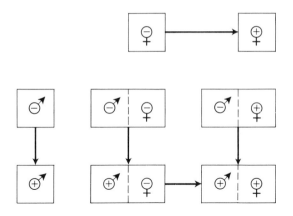

Fig. 7.6. States and transitions of the transmission model used in the present paper. The arrows indicate infectious contacts either within or outside a partnership.

can be considered to be temporarily immune if the male partner belongs to the class with low rates of partner change. Males with a high rate of partner change can infect themselves through occasional contacts with prostitutes. Thus a pair consisting of two susceptibles is transferred into the category of pairs where the male is infected and the female is susceptible. Pairs where one of the two partners is infected and the other is susceptible are transferred into the category of pairs where both are infected at a rate which is the product of the rate of intercourse and the infection probability per act of intercourse.

It was considered essential to list *all* assumptions explicitly so that the results given in the next section can be properly assessed.

4. Results of the simulation

The probability of infection is a very sensitive parameter. If it is taken as 1 per cent the infection cannot maintain itself in the heterosexual population. If, however, it is assumed to be 2 per cent the infection will eventually reach a positive equilibrium in the heterosexual population even if there are no contacts with the homosexual population. Figure 7.7 shows the yearly total number of cases for these two probabilities. The curves with solid symbols refer to the situation where the contacts within the homosexual population stay constant. The curves with the open symbols were obtained by assuming that the contact rate within the homosexual population declines exponentially to one new contact per year. For an infection probability of 1 per cent the total number of cases exponentially approaches zero, whereas for an infection probability of 2 per cent the total number of cases approaches a positive equilibrium. Figures 7.8 and 7.9 show, in addition to the total number of cases, the absolute number of infected individuals and the yearly

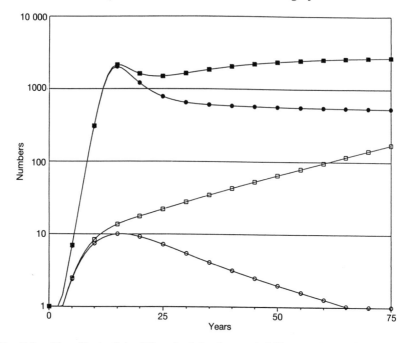

Fig. 7.7. The effect of doubling the infection probability on the total number of cases per year. The circles refer to an infection probability of 1 per cent and the squares refer to an infection probability of 2 per cent. The solid symbols refer to the situation with constant homosexual contact rates and the open symbols refer to the situation where the annual contact rate among homosexuals declines exponentially to unity.

number of new infections for constant homosexual contact rates. For an infection probability of 1 per cent equilibrium is reached after about 30 years, but for an infection probability of 2 per cent the prevalence is still slowly increasing even after 75 years. Table 7.15 shows the effects of doubling the infection probabilities in more detail.

The epidemic is assumed to be started by one homosexual. Table 7.15 specifies the results 75 years after the onset of the epidemic. The population, which has an initial equilibrium size of one million, is constantly replenished by newborns. The fact that after 75 years the total size of the population is only 974 000 and 910 000 for infection probabilities of 1 per cent and 2 per cent respectively, can be interpreted as a reduction in life expectancy due to AIDS. The reduction in life expectancy due to AIDS is 2.6 per cent for an infection probability of 1 per cent but is 9.0 per cent for an infection probability of 2 per cent. This corresponds to an increase by a factor of about 3.5 which is nearly double the increase in the infection probability. There is an even greater increase in the prevalence of infection which is raised from 0.4

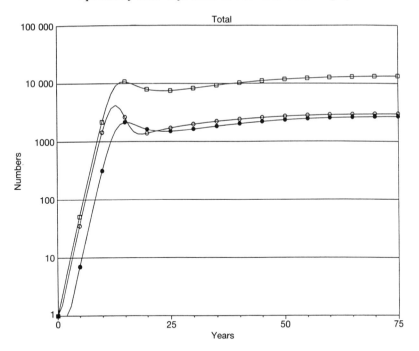

Fig. 7.8. Approach of prevalence (□), infection incidence (○), and incidence of cases (●) to equilibrium for an infection probability of 2 per cent and constant homosexual contact rates.

Table 7.15. The effect of doubling the infection probabilities.

	1	2
Infection probability (per cent)	1	2
Size of total population (thousand)	974	910
Prevalence of infection (per cent)	0.4	2.1
Yearly total incidence of infection (per million)	606	3308
Yearly total incidence of cases (per million)	554	2978
Percentage of males among cases	80	55
Percentage of homosexuals among cases	62	12
Percentage of infections in heterosexual males owing to contacts with prostitutes	22	9
Percentage of infections in females owing to contacts with homosexuals	3	0.5
Prevalence of infection		
Homosexuals (per cent)	78	78
Active prostitutes (per cent)	20	70

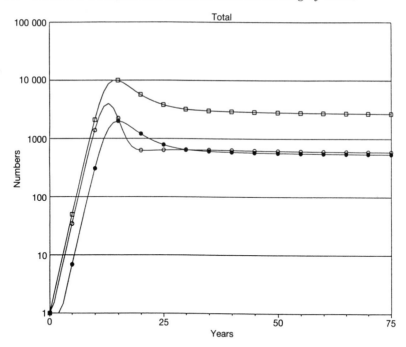

Fig. 7.9.   As for Fig. 7.8 but for an infection probability of 1 per cent.

per cent to 2.1 per cent. Similarly, the yearly total incidence of infection per million and the yearly total incidence of cases per million is increased by more than a factor of 5. The percentage of males among the cases is 80 per cent compared with 55 per cent. As expected the percentage of homosexuals among the cases decreases with an increase in the infection probability but the difference is quite considerable. The model can keep track of the source of infection, which enables us to state that with 1 per cent infection probability 22 per cent of the infections in heterosexual males are due to contacts with prostitutes compared with 9 per cent for an infection probability of 2 per cent. In females the percentage of infections due to contacts with homo-sexuals decreases from 3 per cent to 0.5 per cent. This should not be inter-preted to mean that 3 per cent of the infections in females could be eliminated if there were no contacts with homosexuals. Under the present assumptions the elimination of these contacts would reduce even 100 per cent of the infections in females! The model predicts a 78 per cent equilibrium prevalence in the homosexual population. Among prostitutes the prevalence is increased from 20 per cent to 70 per cent by doubling the infection probability.

Figures 7.10 and 7.11 show the delay in the increase in the number of cases

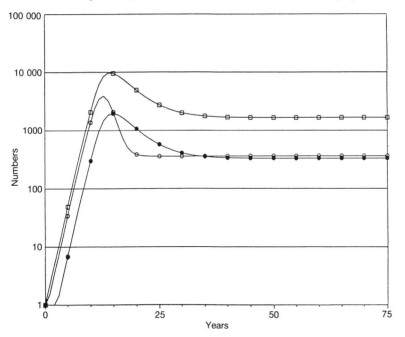

Fig. 7.10. Approach to equilibrium among homosexual men for an infection probability of 2 per cent.

between homosexual and heterosexual men. The curve for heterosexual men rises about 5 years later. In the case of homosexual men prevalence, infection incidence, and case incidence all show a peak which occurs around 15 years after the beginning of the epidemic. In the case of heterosexual men there is initially also an exponential rise which, however, approaches equilibrium without reaching a peak.

If the infection probability and the differential death rate due to AIDS are simultaneously reduced to half their value, a lower death rate due to AIDS is obtained, despite the fact that the infectious period is almost doubled, because a larger proportion will die from other causes (Table 7.16). The reduction in life expectancy declines from 9 per cent to about 5 per cent. However, the prevalence of infection increases from about 2 per cent to 3 per cent. The yearly total incidence of infections decreases slightly, but the yearly total incidence of cases is reduced substantially. The percentage of males and the percentage of homosexuals among the cases is barely affected. The percentage of infections in the heterosexual males as a result of contacts with prostitutes is considerably reduced owing to the overall rise in the prevalence of the infection in the total population. Figure 7.12 shows that the rate of

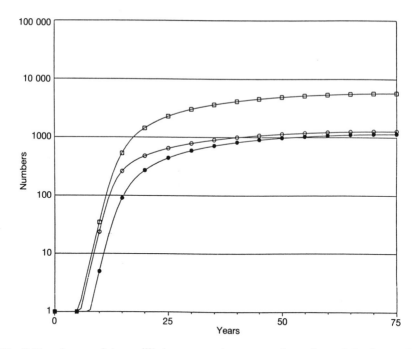

Fig. 7.11.   Approach to equilibrium among heterosexual men for an infection probability of 2 per cent.

Table 7.16.   Effect of simultaneously halving the infection probabilities and the differential death rate due to AIDS.

Infectious period (years)	4.5	8.3
Infection probability (per thousand)	2	1
Size of total population (thousand)	910	949†
Prevalence of infection (per cent)	2.1	3.0
Yearly total incidence of infection (per million)	3308	3212
Yearly total incidence of cases (per million)	2978	2202
Percentage of males among cases	55	56
Percentage of homosexuals among cases	12	14
Percentage of infections in heterosexual males owing to contacts with prostitutes	9	5
Percentage of infections in females owing to contacts with homosexuals	0.5	0.4
Prevalence of infection		
Homosexuals (per cent)	78	76
Active prostitutes (per cent)	70	61

†Values 75 years after begin of the epidemic. The system is not yet in equilibrium.

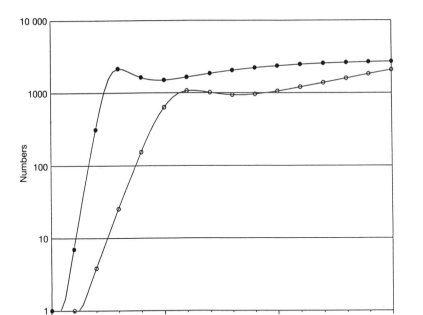

Fig. 7.12. The effect of halving the infection probability h and the differential death rate α due to AIDS on the total number of cases: ●, $h = 0.02$, $\alpha = 0.2$; ○, $h = 0.01$ $\alpha = 0.1$.

Table 7.17. Effect of making contacts with prostitutes 100 per cent safe.

Safety of contacts with prostitutes (per cent)	66.6	100
Size of total population (thousand)	910	979
Prevalence of infection (per cent)	2.1	0.3
Yearly total incidence of infection (per million)	3308	514
Yearly total incidence of cases (per million)	2978	465
Percentage of males among cases	55	86
Percentage of homosexuals among cases	12	73
Percentage of infections in heterosexual males owing to contacts with prostitutes	9	0
Percentage of infections in females owing to contacts with homosexuals	0.5	9
Prevalence of infection		
Homosexuals (per cent)	78	78
Active prostitutes (per cent)	70	0

increase in the total number of cases is lower if the infectious period is longer.

Table 7.17 shows the effect of making all contacts with prostitutes safe. This assumption reduces the reduction in life expectancy from 9 per cent to about 2 per cent. The overall prevalence would be reduced to 0.3 per cent and the incidence of cases from nearly 3,000 to less than 500. The percentage of males among the cases would rise to 86 per cent and the percentage of homosexuals would rise to 73 per cent. The percentage of infections in females resulting from contacts with homosexuals would rise from 0.5 per cent to 9 per cent.

Figure 7.13 shows that the rate of increase in the total number of cases is not affected if the rate of contact of women with bisexual men is either halved or doubled. Figure 7.14 shows the effect reducing the homosexual contacts to a subcritical level or reducing the contacts with prostitutes to zero or a combination of the two. It appears that even in the last-mentioned case the total number of cases would not converge to zero.

Table 7.18 shows the effect of the inactivation of partners of cases. It is assumed that the probability of inactivity after termination of a partnership increases from 2 per cent to 100 per cent if the partnership was terminated by the death of a partner as a result of AIDS. This measure alone would reduce

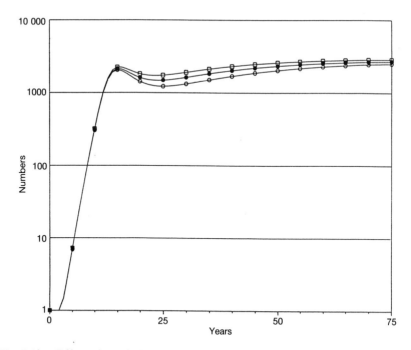

Fig. 7.13.   Effect of modifying the contact rate ϵ with bisexuals on the total number of cases.

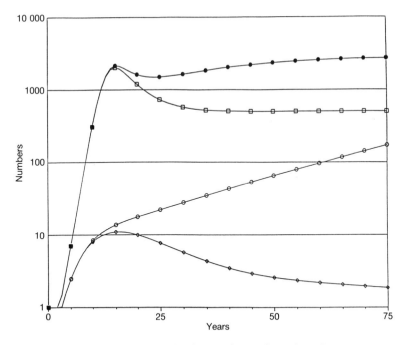

Fig. 7.14. The effect of contact reduction on the total number of cases: ●, no contact reduction; ○, reduction of the contact rate among homosexuals to one partner per year; □, reduction of the infection probability with prostitutes to zero assuming that reduction begins 5 years after the onset of the epidemic and declines at a rate of 14 per cent per year; ◊, combination of the two previous contact reductions.

Table 7.18. Effect of the inactivation of partners of cases.

Probability of inactivation (per cent)	2	100
Size of total population (thousand)	910	963
Prevalence of infection (per cent)	2.1	0.5
Yearly total incidence of infection (per million)	3308	875
Yearly total incidence of cases (per million)	2978	799
Percentage of males among cases	55	71
Percentage of homosexuals among cases	12	43
Percentage of infections in heterosexual males owing to contacts with prostitutes	9	42
Percentage of infections in females owing to contacts with homosexuals	0.5	2.8
Prevalence of infection		
Homosexuals (per cent)	78	78
Active prostitutes (per cent)	70	47

the overall prevalence by a factor of 4, and similarly would reduce the yearly number of cases from about 3000 to 800.

5. Conclusions

(1) It has become clear that the future development of the AIDS epidemic cannot be predicted by simply assuming a continuous exponential rise in the number of cases. It is inevitable that the number of cases per year will eventually reach an equilibrium value which will depend on the contact rates and the characteristics of the virus as they evolve in the near future.

(2) The mathematical model shows that critical parameter values exist below which the infection cannot maintain itself in a population. Therefore the effects of parameter changes are highly non-linear, i.e. a given reduction in a certain parameter will not necessarily lead to the same reduction in a dependent variable. Such critical phenomena often lead to counter-intuitive behaviour of the system. Here the mathematical approach may contribute greatly to the understanding of the observations.

(3) The fact that the number of reported cases implies that at present the heterosexual population is barely affected should not lead to the wrong impression that this will also be true in the future. The model indicates the possibility that a rise similar to that in the homosexual population will occur with a delay of several years. Even if the overall prevalence of the infection in the population stabilizes at about 1 per cent, this could imply several tens of thousands of cases per year in the total population.

(4) At present there is a serious lack of the data required to make these models more realistic. In particular, data on the rates of partner change are crucial for assessment of the situation. Of course, some of the questionnaire studies are unreliable, but the mathematical models could at least be used to provide upper and lower bounds for further studies.

(5) Epidemiological models provide a conceptual framework into which the accumulating data can be integrated and thus can help us to understand the transmission dynamics of the infection. It is to be hoped that it will not be too long before the models can be applied to the evaluation of effective control strategies as in the case of other infectious diseases.

Appendix 7.1.   Equations

Homosexuals

Version 1 (without pair formation):

$$\dot{x}_h = \nu_h - \left(\mu + \frac{h_{11}\beta y_h}{x_h + y_h} \right) x_h$$

$$\dot{y}_h = \frac{h_{11}\beta y_h}{x_h + y_h} x_h - (\alpha + \mu)y_h.$$

Version 2 (with pair formation):

$$\dot{x}_h = \nu_h + 2(\sigma_h + \mu)\left(\frac{p_{h00} + p_{h01}}{2}\right) + \alpha p_{h01} - (2\rho_h + \mu)x_h$$

$$\dot{y}_h = 2(\sigma_h + \mu)\left(\frac{p_{h11} + p_{h01}}{2}\right) + 2\alpha p_{h11} - (2\rho_h + \mu + \alpha)y_h$$

$$\dot{p}_{h00} = \frac{\rho_h x_h^2}{x_h + y_h} - (\sigma_h + 2\mu)p_{h00}$$

$$\dot{p}_{h01} = \frac{2\rho_h x_h y_h}{x_h + y_h} - (\sigma_h + 2\mu + \alpha + h_{11}\varphi_h)p_{h01}$$

$$\dot{p}_{h11} = \frac{\rho_h y_h^2}{x_h + y_h} + h_{11}\varphi_h p_{h01} - (\sigma_h + 2\mu + 2\alpha)p_{h11}.$$

Heterosexuals

$$\dot{x}_{11} = \nu_{11} + (s_{11}\sigma_1 + m_{11}\mu)(p_{100} + p_{101}) + a_{11}\alpha p_{101} -$$
$$- \left\{\mu + \rho_1 + (1-c)\frac{h_{21}\chi_{1s}y_{22}}{x_{22} + y_{22}}\right\}x_{11}$$

$$\dot{y}_{11} = (s_{11}\sigma_1 + m_{11}\mu)(p_{110} + p_{111}) + a_{11}\alpha p_{111} + (1-c)\frac{h_{21}\chi_{1s}y_{22}x_{11}}{x_{22} + y_{22}} -$$
$$- (\mu + \rho_1 + \alpha)y_{11}$$

$$\dot{x}_{12} = \nu_{12} + (s_{12}\sigma_2 + m_{12}\mu)(p_{200} + p_{201}) + a_{12}\alpha p_{201} -$$
$$- \left\{\mu + \rho_2 + (1-c)\frac{h_{21}\chi_{2s}y_{22}}{x_{22} + y_{22}}\right\}x_{12}$$

$$\dot{y}_{12} = (s_{12}\sigma_2 + m_{12}\mu)(p_{210} + p_{211}) + a_{12}\alpha p_{211} + (1-c)\frac{h_{21}\chi_{s2}y_{22}x_{12}}{x_{22} + y_{22}} -$$
$$- (\mu + \rho_2 + \alpha)y_{12}$$

$$\dot{x}_{21} = \nu_{21} + (s_{21}\sigma_1 + m_{21}\mu)(p_{100} + p_{101}) + g\gamma x_{22} + (s_{22}\sigma_2 + m_{22}\mu)(p_{200} + p_{201}) +$$
$$+ a_{21}\alpha p_{110} + a_{22}\alpha p_{210} -$$
$$- \left\{\mu + \frac{\rho_1(x_{11} + y_{11}) + \rho_2(x_{12} + y_{12}) + h_{12}\kappa_{2s}(p_{210} + p_{211}) + h_{12}\epsilon_1 y_h}{x_{21} + y_{21}}\right\}x_{21}$$

$$\dot{y}_{21} = (s_{21}\sigma_1 + m_{21}\mu)(p_{101} + p_{111}) + (s_{22}\sigma_2 + m_{22}\mu)(p_{200} + p_{201}) + g\gamma y_{22} +$$
$$+ a_{21}\alpha p_{111} + a_{22}\alpha p_{211} + h_{12}\kappa_{2s}\frac{p_{210} + p_{211}}{x_{21} + y_{21}} + \frac{h_{12}\epsilon_1 y_h}{x_{21} + y_{21}} -$$
$$- \left\{\mu + \frac{\rho_1(x_{11} + y_{11}) + \rho_2(x_{12} + y_{12})}{x_{21} + y_{21}} + \alpha\right\}y_{21}$$

$$\dot{x}_{22} = \nu_{22} - \left\{ \mu + \gamma + \right.$$

$$\left. + (1-c)h_{12} \frac{\chi_{1s}y_{11} + \chi_{2s}y_{12} + \chi_{1p}(p_{110}+p_{111}) + \chi_{2p}(p_{210}+p_{211}) + \epsilon_2 y_h}{x_{22} + y_{22}} \right\} x_{22}$$

$$\dot{y}_{22} = (1-c)h_{12}x_{22} \frac{\chi_{1s}y_{11} + \chi_{2s}y_{12} + \chi_{1p}(p_{110}+p_{111}) + \chi_{2p}(p_{210}+p_{211}) + \epsilon_2 y_h}{x_{22} + y_{22}} -$$

$$- (\mu + \gamma + \alpha)y_{22}$$

$$\dot{v}_{11} = (1-a_{11})\alpha p_{101} + \{(1-s_{11})\sigma_1 + (1-m_{11})\mu\}(p_{100}+p_{101}) - \mu v_{11}$$

$$\dot{w}_{11} = (1-a_{11})\alpha p_{111} + \{(1-s_{11})\sigma_1 + (1-m_{11})\mu\}(p_{110}+p_{111}) - (\mu+\alpha)w_{11}$$

$$\dot{v}_{12} = (1-a_{12})\alpha p_{201} + \{(1-s_{12})\sigma_2 + (1-m_{12})\mu\}(p_{200}+p_{201}) - \mu v_{12}$$

$$\dot{w}_{12} = (1-a_{12})\alpha p_{211} + \{(1-s_{12})\sigma_2 + (1-m_{12})\mu\}(p_{210}+p_{211}) - (\mu+\alpha)w_{12}$$

$$\dot{v}_{21} = (1-a_{21})\alpha p_{110} + (1-a_{22})\alpha p_{210} + \{(1-s_{21})\sigma_1 + (1-m_{21})\mu\}(p_{100}+p_{110}) +$$

$$+ \{(1-s_{22})\sigma_2 + (1-m_{22})\mu\}(p_{200}+p_{210}) - \mu v_{21}$$

$$\dot{w}_{21} = (1-a_{21})\alpha p_{111} + (1-a_{22})\alpha p_{211} + \{(1-s_{21})\sigma_1 + (1-m_{21})\mu\}(p_{101}+p_{111}) +$$

$$+ \{(1-s_{22})\sigma_2 + (1-m_{22})\mu\}(p_{201}+p_{211}) - (\mu+\alpha)w_{21}$$

$$\dot{v}_{22} = (1-g)\gamma x_{22} - \mu v_{22}$$

$$\dot{w}_{22} = (1-g)\gamma y_{22} - (\mu+\alpha)w_{22}$$

$$P = \sum_{i=1}^{2} \sum_{j=0}^{1} \sum_{k=0}^{1} p_{ijk}$$

$$\dot{p}_{100} = \frac{\rho_1 x_{11} x_{21}}{x_{21}+y_{21}} - \left\{ 2\mu + \sigma_1 + \frac{(1-c)h_{21}\chi_{1p}y_{22}}{x_{22}+y_{22}} + \frac{h_{12}\chi_{2p}(p_{210}+p_{211})}{P} \right\} p_{100}$$

$$\dot{p}_{101} = \frac{\rho_1 x_{11} y_{21}}{x_{21}+y_{21}} + \frac{h_{12}\chi_{2p}(p_{210}+p_{211})p_{100}}{P} -$$

$$- \left\{ 2\mu + \sigma_1 + \alpha + h_{21}\varphi + \frac{(1-c)h_{21}\chi_{1p}y_{22}}{x_{22}+y_{22}} \right\} p_{101}$$

$$\dot{p}_{110} = \frac{\rho_1 x_{21} y_{11}}{x_{21}+y_{21}} + \frac{(1-c)h_{21}\chi_{1p}y_{22}p_{100}}{x_{22}+y_{22}} -$$

$$- \left\{ 2\mu + \sigma_1 + \alpha + h_{12}\varphi + \frac{h_{12}\kappa_{2p}(p_{210}+p_{211})}{P} \right\} p_{110}$$

$$\dot{p}_{111} = \frac{\rho_1 y_{11} y_{21}}{x_{21}+y_{21}} + \frac{(1-c)h_{21}\chi_{1p}y_{22}p_{101}}{x_{22}+y_{22}} + \frac{h_{12}\kappa_{2p}(p_{210}+p_{211})p_{110}}{P} +$$

$$+ \varphi(h_{21}p_{101} + h_{12}p_{110}) - (2\mu + \sigma_1 + 2\alpha)p_{111}$$

$$P_1 = \sum_{i=1}^{2} \sum_{j=0}^{1} p_{ij1}$$

$$\dot{p}_{200} = \frac{\rho_2 x_{12} x_{21}}{x_{21}+y_{21}} - \left\{ 2\mu + \sigma_2 + \frac{(1-c)h_{21}\chi_{2p}y_{22}}{x_{22}+y_{22}} + h_{21}\left(\frac{\kappa_{2s}y_{21}}{x_{21}+y_{21}} + \right. \right.$$

$$\left. \left. + \frac{\kappa_{2p}P_1}{P} \right) + \frac{h_{12}\kappa_{2p}(p_{210}+p_{211})}{P} \right\} p_{200}$$

$$\dot{p}_{201} = \frac{\rho_2 x_{12} y_{21}}{x_{21} + y_{21}} + \frac{h_{12}\kappa_{2p}(p_{210} + p_{211})p_{200}}{P} -$$

$$- \left\{ 2\mu + \sigma_2 + \alpha + h_{21}\varphi + \frac{(1-c)h_{21}\chi_{2p}y_{22}}{x_{22} + y_{22}} + h_{21}\left(\frac{\kappa_{2s}y_{21}}{x_{21} + y_{21}} + \right.\right.$$

$$\left.\left. + \frac{\kappa_{2p}P_1}{P} \right) \right\} p_{201}$$

$$\dot{p}_{210} = \frac{\rho_2 x_{21} y_{12}}{x_{21} + y_{21}} + \frac{(1-c)h_{21}\chi_{2p}y_{22}p_{200}}{x_{22} + y_{22}} + h_{21}\left\{ \frac{\kappa_{2s}y_{21}p_{200}}{x_{21} + y_{21}} + \frac{\kappa_{2p}P_1 p_{200}}{P} \right\} -$$

$$- \left\{ 2\mu + \sigma_2 + \alpha + h_{12}\varphi + \frac{h_{12}\kappa_{2p}(p_{210} + p_{211})}{P} \right\} p_{210}$$

$$\dot{p}_{211} = \frac{\rho_2 y_{12} y_{21}}{x_{21} + y_{21}} + \frac{(1-c)h_{21}\chi_{2p}y_{22}p_{201}}{x_{22} + y_{22}} + h_{21}\left\{ \frac{\kappa_{2s}y_{21}p_{201}}{x_{21} + y_{21}} + \frac{\kappa_{2p}P_1 p_{201}}{P} \right\} +$$

$$+ \frac{h_{12}\kappa_{2p}(p_{210} + p_{211})p_{210}}{P} + \varphi(h_{21}p_{201} + h_{12}p_{210}) - (2\mu + \sigma_2 + 2\alpha)p_{211}$$

Appendix 7.2. Model variables

The variables are listed in the same order as the equations.

Homosexuals

x_h Number of single susceptible homosexuals
y_h Number of single infected homosexuals
p_{h00} Number of homosexual pairs with two susceptible partners
p_{h01} Number of homosexual pairs with one susceptible partner and one infected partner
p_{h11} Number of homosexual pairs with two infected partners

Heterosexuals

x_{11} Number of single susceptible males with a low rate of partner change
y_{11} Number of single infected males with a low rate of partner change
x_{12} Number of single susceptible males with a high rate of partner change
y_{12} Number of single infected males with a high rate of partner change
x_{21} Number of single susceptible females with an average rate of partner change
y_{21} Number of single infected females with an average rate of partner change
x_{22} Number of susceptible prostitutes
y_{22} Number of infected prostitutes
v_{11} Number of inactive susceptible males who had a low rate of partner change
w_{11} Number of inactive infected males who had a low rate of partner change
v_{12} Number of inactive susceptible males who had a high rate of partner change
w_{12} Number of inactive infected males who had a high rate of partner change
v_{21} Number of inactive susceptible females who had an average rate of partner change

w_{21} Number of inactive infected females who had an average rate of partner change

v_{22} Number of inactive susceptible prostitutes

w_{22} Number of inactive infected prostitutes

p_{100} Number of heterosexual pairs with a low rate of partner change and both partners susceptible

p_{101} Number of heterosexual pairs with a low rate of partner change, a susceptible male partner, and an infected female partner

p_{110} Number of heterosexual pairs with a low rate of partner change, an infected male partner, and a susceptible female partner

p_{111} Number of heterosexual pairs with a low rate of partner change and both partners infected

p_{200} Number of heterosexual pairs with a high rate of partner change and both partners susceptible

p_{201} Number of heterosexual pairs with a high rate of partner change, a susceptible male partner, and an infected female partner

p_{210} Number of heterosexual pairs with a high rate of partner change, an infected male partner, and a susceptible female partner

p_{211} Number of heterosexual pairs with a high rate of partner change and both partners infected

Appendix 7.3.   Model parameters

Symbol	Definition	Value
ν_h	Rate at which homosexuals enter the population per year	375
μ	Death rate of an individual per year	0.02
h_{11}	Probability that one sexual contact between a susceptible and an infected homosexual leads to an infection	0.1
β	Rate per year at which homosexuals have single contacts with new partners	10
α	Additional death rate per year of infected individuals	0.2, 0.1
σ_h	Separation rate of homosexual pairs	—
ρ_h	Rate per year at which single homosexuals form pairs	—
φ_h	Rate per year of sexual contact between partners of a homosexual pair	—
ν_{11}	Rate per year at which single susceptible males with a low rate of partner change enter the population	6412.5
s_{11}	Probability that a male with a low rate of	0.98

	partner change stays active after separation	
σ_1	Separation rate per year of a partnership by a male with a low rate of partner change	0.1
m_{11}	Probability that a male with a low rate of partner change stays active after his partner has died from a cause other than AIDS	0.98
a_{11}	Probability that a male with a low rate of partner change stays active after his partner has died as a result of AIDS	0.98, 0
ρ_1	Rate of pair formation by a male with a low rate of partner change per year	1
c	Probability of 'safe sex' during contact with a prostitute	0.66, 1
h_{21}	Probability that one sexual contact of an infected female with a susceptible male leads to an infection	0.01, 0.02
χ_{1s}	Rate per year of contact of single males with a low rate of partner change with prostitutes	0.1
ν_{12}	Rate per year at which males with a high rate of partner change enter the population	712.5
s_{12}	Probability that a male with a high rate of partner change stays active after separation	0.98
σ_2	Separation rate per year of a partnership by a male with a high rate of partner change	1
m_{12}	Probability that a male with a high rate of partner change stays active after his partner has died from a cause other than AIDS	0.98
a_{12}	Probability that a male with a high rate of partner change stays active after his partner has died as a result of AIDS	0.98, 0
ρ_2	Rate per year of pair formation by a male with a high rate of partner change	3
χ_{2s}	Rate per year of contact of single males with a high rate of partner change with prostitutes	5
ν_{21}	Rate per year at which single females with an average rate of partner change enter the population	7492.58
s_{21}	Probability that a female stays active after separation from a male with a low rate of partner change	0.98
m_{21}	Probability that a female stays active after her partner with a low rate of partner change has died from a cause other than AIDS	0.98
g	Probability that a prostitute joins the group of	0

	single active females after becoming inactive as a prostitute	
γ	Rate per year at which a prostitute becomes inactive	0.1
s_{22}	Probability that a female stays active after separation from a male with a high rate of partner change	0.98
m_{22}	Probability that a female stays active after her partner with a high rate of partner change has died from a cause other than AIDS	0.98
a_{21}	Probability that a female stays active after her partner with a low rate of partner change has died as a result of AIDS	0.98, 0
a_{22}	Probability that a female stays active after her partner with a high rate of partner change has died as a result of AIDS	0.98, 0
h_{12}	Probability that one sexual contact of an infected male with a susceptible female leads to an infection	0.01, 0.02
κ_{2s}	Rate per year of contact of a paired male with a high rate of partner change with single females	0
ϵ_1	Rate per year at which a homosexual man has contacts with single females	0.1, 0.2, 0.4
ν_{22}	Rate per year at which prostitutes enter the population	7.5
χ_{1p}	Rate per year at which a paired male with a low rate of partner change has contacts with prostitutes	0
χ_{2p}	Rate per year at which a paired male with a high rate of partner change has contacts with prostitutes	0.5
ϵ_2	Rate per year at which a homosexual has contacts with prostitutes	0.5
κ_{2p}	Rate per year at which a paired male with a high rate of partner change has contacts with paired females	0
φ	Rate per year of sexual contact within a heterosexual pair	100

Acknowledgments

The author would like to thank Mr J. Meyer for his efficient support in programming the present model and producing the graphical output.

References

Anderson, R.M., May, R.M., Medley, G.F., and Johnson, A.M. (1986). A preliminary study of the transmission dynamics of the human immunodeficiency virus (HIV) the causative agent of AIDS. *IMA Journal of Mathematics Applied in Biology and Medicine*, **3**, 229–63.

Bailey, N.T.J. and Estreicher, J. (1987). Epidemic description and public health control with special reference to influenza and AIDS. In Proc. 1st World Congress Bernoulli Soc., Vol. 2, VNU Science Press, 507–16.

Cochran, W.G., Mosteller, F., and Tukey, J.W. (1954). *Statistical problems of the Kinsey Report on sexual behaviour in the human male*. The American Statistical Association, Washington, DC.

Dannecker, M. and Reiche, R. (1974). *Der gewöhnliche Homosexuelle. Eine soziologische Untersuchung über männliche Homosexuelle in der Bundesrepublik*. Fischer Verlag, Frankfurt.

Dietz, K. and Schenzle, D. (1985). Mathematical models for infectious disease statistics. In *A celebration of statistics* (eds A.C. Atkinson and S.E. Fienberg), pp. 167–204. Springer, New York.

Dörner, D. (1986). Ein Simulationsprogramm für die Ausbreitung von AIDS. *Memorandum No. 40, Projekt 'Systemdenken', DFG 200/5*. Lehrstuhl Psychologie II, Universität Bamberg.

van Druten, J.A.M., de Boo, Th., Jager, J.C., Heisterkamp, S.H. Coutinho, R.A., and Ruitenberg, E.J. (1986). AIDS prediction and intervention. *Lancet* i, 852–3.

Eichner, K. and Habermehl, W. (1978). *Der RALF-Report. Das Sexualverhalten der Deutschen*. Hoffman und Campe, Hamburg.

Hethcote, H.W. and Yorke, J.A. (1984). Gonorrhea transmission dynamics and control. *Lecture Notes in Biomathematics* **56**.

Kiessling, D., Stannat, S., Schedel, I., and Deicher, H. (1986). Überlegungen und Hochrechnungen zur Epidemiologie des 'Acquired Immunodeficiency Syndrome' in der Bundesrepublik Deutschland. *Infection* **14**, 217–22.

Knox, E.G. (1986). A transmission model for AIDS. *European Journal of Epidemiology* **2**, 165–77.

Koch, M.G. (1985). *Vår Framtid?* Svenska Carnegie Institutet, Stockholm.

Kolb, I. (1980). *Das Kreuz mit der Liebe*. Gruner und Jahr, Hamburg.

Martini, E. (1928). Betrachtungen zur Epidemiologie der Malaria und der Syphilis. *Dermatologische Wochenschrift* **19**, 640–3.

Pickering, J., Wiley, J.A., Padian, N.S., Lieb, L.E., Echenberg, D.F., and Walker, J. (1986). Modeling the incidence of acquired immunodeficiency syndrome (AIDS) in San Francisco, Los Angeles, and New York. *Mathematical Modelling* **7**, 661–88.

Ross, R. (1911). *The prevention of malaria* (2nd edn). Murray, London.

8

Modelling the AIDS epidemic

E.G. Knox

1. Application of models

We all prefer facts to projections, but facts exist only in the past. Planners are concerned with the future, where there are no facts, and so facts are no use to them unless they can project the observations towards the future. Extrapolation from the known towards the unknown *always* demands that we use a model. There is no other route. We can use physical, mathematical, computer-simulation, or diagrammatic (iconic) models—but we have to use a model of some kind.

2. What do we need to predict about AIDS?

(i) What will be the peak prevalence of HIV infection, the peak incidence of new HIV infections, and the peak incidence of AIDS? What will the care of AIDS cost?

(ii) How long will it take to get there? What will be the position one planning cycle from now? How many AIDS doubling times are there to a planning cycle?

(iii) Is HIV infection self-sustaining in the heterosexual population?

(iv) What will be the effect of a general modification of sexual behaviour?

(v) What will be the effect of selective behaviour change in response to targeted health education?

(vi) What will be the effect of a treatment which prolongs the health and sexual mobility of infectious individuals?

(vii) How effective will a vaccine be? Must we vaccinate everyone or can it be targeted to subsets of the population (for example, high risk groups alone, or those presenting with gonorrhoea, or only boys)?

(viii) What if a vaccine is at first only 50 per cent (or x per cent) effective? How should we deploy it? If its effects fade in time, is it better to deploy a limited supply across the whole population or to give it repeatedly to high risk groups?

We are likely to face any or all of these problems at short notice within the next few months and years.

3. What else is a model good for besides predicting the future?

(i) It specifies quite exactly the data necessary for achieving accurate prediction. Therefore we know how to design our research enquiries.

(ii) If the data are not available, but can be guessed, it permits interim conditional predictions: *If* this, *then* that. . . .

(iii) It allows us to conduct a 'sensitivity analysis' to discover which of our factual uncertainties are crucial, where a guess might do, and where research is urgent.

4. Available models

The course of the AIDS epidemic can be predicted through one or more of the following mechanisms:

(i) by extrapolating the points on the approximately logarithmic curve of increase of AIDS, backed up by a similar procedure for newly diagnosed cases of HIV infection;

(ii) by applying the current understanding of the natural history of HIV infections to the measured (or estimated) pool of those who are HIV positive but have not yet developed AIDS;

(iii) by watching progress in countries with analogous social structures which are already further down the epidemic path (e.g. USA);

(iv) by constructing theoretical (mathematical/computer-simulation) models of the spread of the disease, validating the outputs of the model against available population data, and subsequently extrapolating to the future.

The first three methods are valid for the first three or four doubling times beyond the present. The current doubling time is about 10 months. Method (ii) is possibly valid for a little longer: the median time to onset of AIDS following infection is now thought to be about 6 years. However, the disease cannot go on doubling for ever and must level off somewhere. Where? Theoretical models provide the only prospects of longer-term projections and solutions to questions of these kinds. The projections will be uncertain at first, but will sharpen as the quantitative tolerances of the parameters are narrowed through the acquisition of new data. Such models are also necessary for estimating the probable effects of treatments and vaccines upon the course of the epidemic before they become available in order to declare the terms in which their efficacies must be specified by manufacturers if we are to use them effectively and to devise optimal deployments during an initial period of shortage. These predictions also form the necessary basis of any long-term economic projections and of planning decisions for the provision of health-care services. Such models also allow us to predict the effects of behavioural changes following health education programmes (once the consequential behavioural changes have been measured) and to predict the effects of targeted deployments of health education towards particular sexual-behavioural groups.

5. An equilibrium model

Equilibrium models are widely used in all branches of science. The classical equilibrium models used in epidemiology are usually termed 'mass-action' models. They depend upon the proposition that the numbers of cases about to occur are proportional to both the current number of susceptibles and the current number of infectious persons. If we represent the current proportion of infectious persons as p and the proportion of susceptibles as $1 - p$, the rate of growth of the epidemic is proportional to $p(1 - p)$. This rate also depends on the contact rate a between infectious and susceptible persons and upon the risk t of transfer of infection when an infectious person comes into contact with a susceptible person. The epidemic then grows in proportion to $atp(1 - p)$.

If infectious people recover from their disease at a rate of D per year, the numbers recovering each year are represented as pD. (In the case of AIDS, recovery from the infectious state is through death, and through replacement by a new susceptible!) The disease will settle out at a steady level when the growth rate is exactly equal to the 'recovery' rate, i.e. when

$$atp(1 - p) - pD = 0.$$

This can be simplified to give an expression for the prevalence $\bar{p}$ at equilibrium:

$$\bar{p} = 1 - \frac{D}{at}.$$

If $D > at$, then the disease will disappear; if $0 < D < at$, then the disease achieves equilibrium, i.e. $0 < \bar{p} < 1$.

6. Complications

The expressions set out above are satisfactory for asexual transmission of a disease such as plantar warts. For heterosexually transmitted diseases the expressions are more complicated and we have to designate values for atp and D separately for each sex. If we use a_1, t_1, D_1, and p_1 to represent the values for males, and a_2, t_2, D_2, and p_2 to represent the values in females, the equilibrium values work out as

$$\bar{p}_1 = \frac{(a_1 t_1)(a_2 t_2) - D_1 D_2}{(a_2 t_2)\{(a_1 t_1) + D_1\}}$$

$$\bar{p}_2 = \frac{(a_1 t_1)(a_2 t_2) - D_1 D_2}{(a_1 t_1)\{(a_2 t_2) + D_2\}}.$$

For a sexually transmitted disease to survive in the population the (common) numerators of these two equations must be positive; otherwise, the disease disappears. With some minor simplifications (i.e. $a_1 = a_2$ and $D_1 = D_2$) this is the same as saying that, for the disease to survive, a must be greater than $D/(t_1 t_2)^{1/2}$.

D for AIDS is about 0.1, because the disease is infectious for about 10 years (i.e. $1/D$). If we assume that the risk to a susceptible female from an infectious partner during the whole of the partnership is about 0.1, and if we assume that the risk to a susceptible male from an infectious female is about 0.025, then we calculate that a has to be greater than 2 for the disease to survive. In other words, an HIV-self-sustaining stratum of the population will be one which takes new partners more frequently than twice per year. This may not be the *actual* figure, and we are very short of accurate information on the appropriate values for t_1 and t_2. The point to be emphasized is that this provides a critical value which will determine whether the disease survives in the heterosexual population (through sexual transmission alone) or whether it does not.

All our theoretical evidence, and much of our recent factual evidence, suggests that the critical value is well within the current range of behaviour.

7. More complications

AIDS is not simply a heterosexually transmitted disease but passes between homosexuals, between bisexuals and heterosexuals, between heterosexuals, between mother and foetus, and between drug users who share syringes and needles. There are *many* different kinds of pair contacts, and not simply the male–female contacts which we usually consider in the common sexually transmitted diseases. The transmission risks are also asymmetric, being greater as a rule for one member of the pair (if the other is infectious) than the other way round. Third, through the medium of female and homosexual prostitution, some of these partnerships are highly asymmetric with respect to a, and one member of the pair is much more promiscuous as well as much less 'abundant' than the other.

These complications take the calculations beyond the domain of simple algebra and require the construction of a computer program. This has been done. A range of different projections were based upon different estimated values for the parameters. These outcomes have been reported (Knox 1986).

8. Results

These enquiries predict that the equilibrium prevalence of HIV in the UK will attain an equilibrium prevalence in the region of 12 per thousand sexually active persons, and probably between 8 per 1,000 and 16 per 1,000. This would give rise to between 20 000 and 40 000 deaths from AIDS per year in the UK. Both the projected prevalence of HIV infection and its response to behavioural changes are unevenly distributed in the different behaviour groups. For example, using plausible estimates for a, t, and D, the equilibrium prevalence will reach about 80 per cent in promiscuous male homosexual anal-receptives and about 90 per cent in female prostitutes, whereas in non-promiscuous to not very promiscuous heterosexual males and females the values will be of the order of 1.5–6.5 per cent. The annual incidences of HIV infection will be about one-tenth $(1/D)$ of these values per year, and the incidence of AIDS will be some fraction of that, say 20–60 per cent. There is now some evidence that some of these predictions are proving reasonably accurate.

Modifications of the equilibrium model allow us to project the *rate* at which these equilibrium positions will be approached. In the more promiscuous groups, the equilibrium positions will be reached in 10–15 years, while in the less promiscuous groups the process will take 30 or 40 years, or perhaps even longer. Indeed, projections at this distance reveal the limitations of an equilibrium model. Few people go on changing partners for this period of time, and some groups will never reach their equilibrium values. At this point it becomes necessary to begin to develop *dynamic* models in order to supplement and modify the predictions of the model outlined here. Model experiments with 'successful' health education campaigns—successful in the sense that they altered the rate of partner change by up to 30 per cent—showed that the reductions in prevalence and death rate (within this range) were proportional to the degree to which the behaviour was altered. However, there was little hope, within any reasonable expectation of a behavioural response, that the epidemic would thereby be controlled or the transmission process halted.

The model was also used to predict the population effectiveness of vaccines given to the whole population, or to a fraction of the population, or to fractions of the promiscuous classes alone. These experiments suggested that the situation would indeed be very responsive to a good vaccine, and particularly responsive to a combination of a good vaccine and a good health education campaign. Reductions in the rate of partner change appear to be *more than* proportionately effective in reducing prevalence and incidence when given a 'head start' by a vaccine, even when the vaccine is in short supply and is deployed selectively to high risk groups. Indeed, it is already clear that it a combination of a vaccine *and* a substantial alteration in behaviour patterns will be required if we are to control this epidemic.

References

Knox, E.G. (1986). A transmission model for AIDS. *European Journal of Epidemiology* **2**, 165–177.

9

Interactive simulation as a tool in the decision-making process to prevent HIV incidence among homosexual men in The Netherlands: a proposal

M.G.W. Dijkgraaf, G.J.P. van Griensven, and J.L.A. Geurts

---

1. Irrational policies

In the absence of a medical solution to the problem of AIDS and without knowing if or when there will be one, a pressing need exists to counter the further spread of HIV among homosexual men by means of political and social measures.[1,2] Several organizations and agencies in The Netherlands are active in this area.[2] Measures include AIDS leaflets, safe-sex parties, testing facilities, health education, and the encouragement of condom use. From the perspective of rational decision making, however, questions can be raised about these activities.

Have the basic ideas behind the selection of measures like these been formulated explicitly?
Have all possible measures been discussed?
Have all possible effects of the measures been taken into account?

Up to now measures have generally been selected on intuitive grounds without full account being taken of the questions listed above. Most reasoning has taken a simple form such as: 'If condoms prevent transmission of HIV, then people should start using condoms'. However, what exactly can be expected to be the outcome of a campaign urging the use of condoms? Will this campaign be more effective than other measures?

Policy-making is clearly a difficult task. At least four areas exist in which policy makers are confronted with difficulties.[3]

2. Problem areas

The scientific area. Many aspects of the behavioural and physical system of forces causing the explosive spread of AIDS are still unknown. However, current knowledge clearly indicates that this system is very complicated. Many variables interact at different levels (micro, meso, and macro), and the relations between the variables are often complex (showing non-linearities, delays, and feedback). As a result, although it may be possible to sort out the different variables affected by particular preventive measures, it is unlikely that it will be possible to forecast the final changes in these variables because of their dynamic interactions. Thus some effects of preventive actions may be opposite to those expected. For instance, forced closure of gay saunas and bars in order to reduce the number of risky sexual contacts may have a number of unexpected side-effects. One of these is that the break-up of more or less closed circuits of intensively interacting individuals might lead to a long-term acceleration of the diffusion of HIV, because members of these circuits will spread through the total population at risk, thereby increasing the probability of contact between an uninfected and an infected individual.

The economic area. The finance available for preventive measures is determined by economics, which thus exerts an external influence on the selection of measures. This must be taken into account.

The social–political–ethical area. Measures must be taken in an ethical, social, and political context. However, this may change over time and influence reactions to measures being taken or under consideration. For instance, when the AIDS epidemic becomes more threatening to the population at large, society may put pressure on policy makers to implement more restrictive preventive measures than they are professionally willing to adopt.

The time-scale. The speed of diffusion of HIV puts pressure on policy makers to develop and implement measures as soon as possible.

Since policy makers have to deal with the difficulties and pressures in each of these different but interrelated areas, it comes as no surprise that they take decisions based on intuition and their experience in the field. However, the process of policy making can be rationalized and put on a more explicit level than it is at present. As a result policy makers will have a firmer grip on the difficulties encountered. We propose a policy-supporting tool which will enable the policy-making process to be rationalized.

3. The tool

The policy-supporting tool should satisfy two important demands. First, it should integrate existing knowledge of the behavioural and physical system of forces which causes the disease to spread. At the same time it should indicate the current state of discussion and understanding of preventive measures. As these are still at an early stage, the second property of the tool should be to trigger discussions among policy makers so that they can exchange ideas as to the best way of proceeding in this complex and uncertain situation.

A simulation type of predecision tool can help with this problem. The human mind is not always capable of handling the complex interactions in a set of variables over a period of time.[3-5] A formal model representing the current state of knowledge and programmed for a computer can be a powerful, although hypothetical, aid to elucidation of the dynamic effects of particular preventive measures. For example, it is not uncommon in situations of this type for the short-term consequences of a measure to be different from the long-term consequences. Simulation with an appropriate internal structure and time horizon would reveal such differences. An additional advantage of a formal model is its contribution to the accuracy of the discussion. A formal model forces the model builder and the participating policy maker to give a precise description of what is meant by a particular preventive measure and how it is likely to influence behaviour. The advantages of a formal model can be summarized as follows:[6]

> an exact description of assumptions and relations is required; logical contra-dictions are avoided;
> gaps in information are revealed by the requirement of precise specification;
> fast low-budget simulation experiments, which enable the consequences of assumptions to be assessed easily, can be performed;
> more than one strategy can be evaluated efficiently;
> the model cannot be changed without conscious manipulation.

The method chosen is called *interactive simulation*. It contains the formal model and the procedure encouraging policy makers to discuss the model, the outcomes of the simulation experiments, and their conclusions regarding the effectiveness and desirability of particular policy measures. Interactive simulation has already been used to elucidate and explore heroin policy[7] and social security policy.[4] There is another reason for this choice. Interactive simulation is very suitable for *instruction and education* purposes. Since the model gives a relatively simplified view of the problem of AIDS and can be displayed using a microcomputer, groups of lay people and persons at risk can be introduced to many aspects of AIDS and the diffusion of the virus.

4. The model

Figure 9.1 shows a simple model in which various symbols are used. These symbols are defined in Appendix 9.1. Appendix 9.2 shows the basic equations of the model written in DYNAMO.[8]

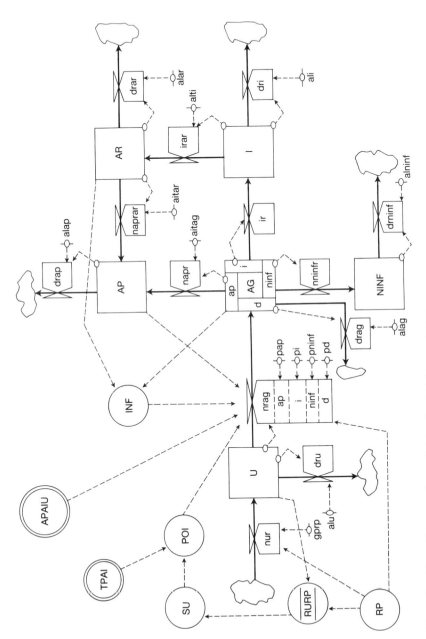

Fig. 9.1. Flow diagram of a model for the incidence of HIV.

The model is partly based on data from recently published studies[1,9,10] and will be our point of reference at the start of the interactive simulation. It will then be changed by redefinition of the central concepts and formulation of new extensions. This will be a continuous process as the interactive simulation program runs. It is not necessary to give a detailed description of the basic model, and so for simplicity less important aspects are not considered here.

Levels, symbolized by squares, represent numbers of persons in different categories. The six squares shown represent a total of nine categories (for simplicity one of them represents four categories). These nine categories are discrete groups in the natural history of HIV infection. Uninfected persons (U) become infected and start producing antigen (AG). Some of them (AGAP) will develop AIDS symptoms (AP) directly and others (AGI) will develop them indirectly, i.e. after going through stages in which antigen disappears (I) and reappears (AR). Persons not developing AIDS symptoms will either become non-infectious (AGNINF → NINF) or will leave the model as a result of death from natural causes at the antigen-production stage (AGD → DRAG), antigen-disappearance stage (I → DRI), or antigen-reappearance stage (AR → DRAR).

Rates, symbolized by 'taps', represent numbers of persons moving from one level to another in the direction indicated by the arrows within a specified period of time. Only rates can change levels. The most important rate is the one representing HIV incidence (NRAG or new rate of infected persons; antigen productive). This incidence depends on the following (see the broken arrows pointing to NRAG, except for those on the right (PAP, PI, PNINF, and PD)):

(a) the number of uninfected persons (U);
(b) the average number of partners with whom uninfected persons have risky contact, e.g. anal intercourse (APAIU);
(c) the probability of contacting an infectious partner, which is equal to the number of infectious persons (INF) divided by the number of persons in the population at risk (RP) excluding the AIDS patients (AP);
(d) the probability of infection (POI).

The probability of infection itself depends on the transmission potential of the risky contact (TPAI) and the susceptibility of the uninfected group of persons (SU), which varies with the ratio (RURP) of the number of uninfected persons (U) to the number of persons in the population at risk (RP).

During interactive simulation preventive measures will be linked to the variables influencing HIV incidence (NRAG). For instance, widespread encouragement of condom use and dissemination of information will be linked to the probability of infection (POI) which in turn influences HIV incidence (NRAG).

Finally, it should be noted that several assumptions have been made in the construction of this basic model. Although these assumptions may be temporary as a result of the game process, we list the most important:

no time constant is given for the progress of persons classed as AGI and AGNINF to I and NINF respectively, because the change is almost instantaneous in the time horizon of the model;
infectious persons (INF) are those with antigen in their body fluids (AGAP, AGI, AGNINF, AGD, and AR); AIDS patients do not take part in risky contacts either because they are unable to do so or because they know the risks to which they expose their partner;
homogeneous mixing.

Appendix 9.1

Symbol	Name	Explanation
	Level	State of affairs (variable), e.g. number of AIDS patients in The Netherlands
	Rate	Stream (variable), e.g. new AIDS patients in last month
	Source	Level of no relevance to the model, e.g. total number of dead non-infectious persons
	Auxiliary	Variable which helps to link level and rate, e.g. number of infectious persons
	Table function	The relation is expressed by a table and not analytically, e.g. ratio of uninfected persons to all persons in population at risk
	External	This variable is external to the model
	Constant	For example, growth percentage of risk population
	Stream of persons	
	Stream of information	For example, causal links

Appendix 9.2   Model for the incidence of HIV

```
*
note
L      U.K. = U.J + DT*(NUR.JK – NRAGD.JK – NRAGNI.JK –
X            NRAGI.JK – NRAGAP.JK – DRU.JK)
N      U = ?
note      U       — number of infected persons
note      NUR     — new rate of uninfected persons
note      NRAGD   — new rate of infected persons (antigen
note                productive) (HIV incidence), no further
note                development
note      NRAGNI — new rate of infected persons (antigen
note                productive) (HIV incidence), development
note                of non-infectiousness at later date
note      NRAGI   — new rate of infected persons (antigen
note                productive) (HIV incidence), indirect
note                development of AIDS symptoms at later
note                date
note      NRAGAP— new rate of infected persons (antigen
note                productive) (HIV incidence), direct
note                development of AIDS symptoms at later
note                date
note      DRU     — death rate of uninfected persons
R      NUR.KL = RP.K*GPRP
C      GPRP = ?
note      GPRP    — percentage growth of the population at risk
note      RP      — number of persons in the population at risk
R      NRAGD.KL = (POI.K*U.K*APAIU.K*INF.K*PD)/
X      (RP.K – AP.K)
C      PD = ?
note      POI     — probability of infection
note      APAIU   — average number of partners, anal
note                intercourse for uninfected persons
note      INF     — number of infectious persons sexually active
note      PD      — percentage of infected persons (antigen
note                productive) with no further development
note      AP      — number of AIDS patients
R      NRAGNI.KL = (POI.K*U.K*APAIU.K*INF.K*PNINF)/
X      (RP.K – AP.K)
C      PNINF = ?
note      PNINF   — percentage of infected persons (antigen
note                productive) developing non-infectiousness
```

note	at later date
R	NRAGI.KL = (POI.K*U.K*APAIU.K*INF.K*PI)/ (RP.K – AP.K)
C	PI = ?
note	PI — percentage of infected persons (antigen
note	productive) indirectly developing AIDS
note	symptoms at later date
R	NRAGAP.KL = (POI.K*U.K*APAIU.K*INF.K*PAP)/
X	(RP.K – AP.K)
C	PAP = ?
note	PAP — percentage of infected persons (antigen
note	productive) directly developing AIDS
note	symptoms at later date
R	DRU.KL = U.K/ALU
C	ALU = ?
note	ALU — average life expectancy of uninfected
note	persons (in DT)
L	AGD.K = AGD.J + DT*(NRAGD.JK – DRAG.JK)
N	AGD = ?
R	DRAG.KL = AGD.K/ALAG
C	ALAG = ?
note	AGD — number of infected persons (antigen
note	productive) with no further development
note	DRAG — death rate of infected persons (antigen
note	productive)
note	ALAG — average life expectancy of antigen-
note	productive persons (in DT)
L	AGNINF.K = AGNINF.J + DT*(NRAGNI.JK – NNINFR.JK)
N	AGNINF = ?
R	NNINFR.KL = AGNINF.K
note	AGNINF — number of infected persons (antigen
note	productive) developing non-infectiousness
note	at later date
note	NNINFR — new rate of non-infectious persons
L	AGI.K = AGI.J + DT*(NRAGI.JK – IR.JK)
N	AGI = ?
R	IR.KL = AGI.K
note	AGI — number of infected persons (antigen
note	productive) indirectly developing AIDS
note	symptoms at later date
note	IR — rate of infected persons (antigen absent)
L	AGAP.K = AGAP.J + DT*(NRAGAP.JK – NAPR.JK)
N	AGAP = ?
R	NAPR.KL = AGAP.K/AITAG

C	AITAG = ?
note	AGAP — number of infected persons (antigen
note	productive) directly developing AIDS
note	symptoms at later date
note	NAPR — new rate of AIDS patients (antigen
note	productive)
note	AITAG — average incubation time for antigen-
note	productive persons (in DT)
L	NINF.K = NINF.J + DT*(NNINFR.JK – DRNINF.JK)
N	NINF = ?
R	DRNINF.KL = NNINF.K/ALNINF
C	ALNINF = ?
note	NINF — number of non-infectious persons
note	DRNINF — death rate of non-infectious persons
note	ALNINF — average life expectancy of non-infectious
note	persons (in DT)
L	I.K = I.J + DT*(IR.JK – DRI.JK – IRAR.JK)
N	I = ?
R	DRI.KL = I.K/ALI
C	ALI = ?
R	IRAR.KL = I.K/ALTI
C	ALTI = ?
note	I — number of infected persons (antigen absent)
note	DRI — death rate of infected persons (antigen
note	absent)
note	IRAR — rate of infected persons (antigen
note	reproductive)
note	ALI — average life expectancy infected persons
note	(antigen absent) (in DT)
note	ALTI — average latency time of infected persons
note	(antigen absent) (in DT)
L	AR.K = AR.J + DT*(IRAR.JK – DRAR.JK – NAPRAR.JK)
N	AR = ?
R	DRAR.KL = AR.K/ALAR
C	ALAR = ?
R	NAPRAR.KL = AR.K/AITAR
C	AITAR = ?
note	AR — number of infected persons (antigen
note	reproductive)
note	DRAR — death rate of infected persons (antigen
note	reproductive)
note	NAPRAR— new rate of AIDS patients (antigen
note	reproductive)

note	ALAR	— average life expectancy persons (antigen
note		reproductive) (in DT)
note	AITAR	— average incubation time for persons
note		(antigen reproductive) (in DT)
L	AP.K = AP.J + DT*(NAPR.JK + NAPRAR.JK – DRAP.JK)	
N	AP = ?	
R	DRAP.KL = AP.K/ALAP	
C	ALAP = ?	
note	AP	— number of AIDS patients
note	DRAP	— death rate of AIDS patients
note	ALAP	— average life expectancy of AIDS patients
note		(in DT)
A	POI.K = SU.K*TPAI.K	
note	SU	— susceptibility of uninfected persons
note	TPAI	— transmission potential of anal intercourse
A	APAIU.K: variable depending on future extensions of the	
X		model, but for the first set of simulations set at a
X		particular value
A	INF.K = AGD.K + AGNINF.K + AGI.K + AGAP.K + AR.K	
A	RP.K = U.K + AGD.K + AGNINF.K + AGI.K + AGAP.K +	
X	NINF.K + I.K + AR.K + AP.K	
A	SU.K = TABLE(SUT,RURP.K,?,?,?)	
T	SUT = ?/?/?/?/?/?	
note	RURP	— ratio of number of uninfected persons to
note		number of persons in risk population
A	RURP.K = U.K/RP.K	
A	TPAI.K: see APAIU.K	

References

1 van Griensven, G.J.P., Tielman, R.A.P., Goudsmit, J., van der Noordaa, J., de Wolf, F., and Coutinho, R.A. (1986). Risikofaktoren en prevalentie van LAV/HTLV III antistoffen bij homoseksuele mannen in Nederland. *Tijdschrift voor Sociale Gezondheidszorg* **64** (4), 100–7.

2 Landelijke beleidscoordinatie AIDS. (1986). *Voorlichting en preventie in het kader van AIDS*. Nota, Amsterdam.

3 Geurts, J.L.A. (1983). Sociale planning, systeemdenken en simulate. *Systemica* **3** (2/3), 93–115.

4 Geurts, J.L.A., van Griensven, G.J.P., Gubbels, J.W., and Vennix, J.A.M. (1985). The social security system in the Netherlands. An interactive simulation. *Simulation and Games* **16** (3), 289–310.

5 Forrester, J.W. (1961). *Industrial dynamics*. MIT Press, Cambridge, Mass.

6 Smits, R.E.H.M. (1983). Systeemdynamica en beleidsgericht onderzoek. *Systemica* **3** (2/3), 117–58.

7   Levin, G., Roberts, E.B., and Hirsch, G.B. (1977). *The persistent poppy. A computer-aided search for heroin policy*. Ballinger, Cambridge, Mass.

8   Richardson, G.P. and Pugh, A.L., III. (1981). *Introduction to system dynamics modeling with DYNAMO*. MIT Press, Cambridge, Mass.

9   Coutinho, R.A., Goudsmit, J., Paul, D.A., de Wolf. F., Lange, J., van der Noordaa, J., and the Dutch AIDS Study Group. (1987). The natural history of HIV infection in homosexual men. *Ann. Inst. Pasteur/Virol.* **138**, 67–74.

10 Goudsmit, J., Paul, D.A., Lange, J.M.A., *et al.* (1986). Expression of human immunodeficiency virus antigen (HIV-ag) in serum and cerebrospinal fluid during acute and chronic infection. *Lancet* **ii**, 177–80.

10

The prognostic analysis of the AIDS epidemic: mathematical modelling and computer simulation

J.J. Gonzalez, M.G. Koch, D. Dörner,
J. L'age-Stehr, M. Myrtveit, and L. Vavik

1. Introduction

It is well known that AIDS is caused by a new lentivirus called HIV (Barré-Sinoussi *et al.* 1983; Karpas 1983; Popovic *et al.* 1984; Levy *et al.* 1984). When a new lentivirus spreads insidiously in a sufficiently homogeneous population (a compartment), there is an initial stage where the following two conditions are approximately satisfied: the number of virus carriers is very small compared with the number of susceptibles, and the factors governing transmission of the disease are roughly the same during the time interval considered. In such a case the average number of virus carriers grows exponentially (Gonzalez and Koch 1986, 1987). We refer to this initial stage, when the number of virus carriers in a compartment behaves exponentially, as the *exponential phase*.

Turning now to the recorded AIDS cases, it is well known that in most countries the AIDS epidemic follows a quasi-exponential law with an apparent gradual decline of the growth rate which begins quite early (Downs *et al.* 1987, 1988; Tillett and McEvoy 1986). As measured by the doubling time for AIDS patients, the growth rate is initially of the order of 5–7 months, and is 8–12 months 3–4 years later. Many people would assume this slowing down of the growth rate to be due to changes of behaviour of risk groups and to prophylactic measures, and possibly also to the depletion of subpopulations in the sense that reinfection of a virus carrier does not increase the size of the epidemic. In the next section we present evidence that in numerous countries (in fact, in all countries we have investigated) most or all of the apparent decline in the growth rate in the recorded AIDS cases within the first 3–6 years of the epidemic can be explained as a spurious effect due to a so-called (onset) *transient*. In other words, in all countries investigated good agreement with recorded AIDS cases is obtained with a purely exponential law for the number of virus carriers during an initial stage with a duration of 3–6 years. Additional evidence for this claim can be given through comparison of an exponential law for the virus spread with a logistic curve: for the parameters in question the logistic curve for the countries investigated does not differ significantly from an exponential curve in the initial stage (Gonzalez and Koch 1986, 1987, 1988). The duration of the initial exponential phase depends on the characteristics of the national epidemic, and hence it is quite different from country to country. The typical extent of the exponential phase is the first 3–6 years of the visible AIDS epidemic.

To avoid misunderstanding, we emphasize that no claim is made that the major part of the decline in the growth rate of the epidemic *after* the initial stage can be explained as an exponential law for the spread of the virus plus superposed transient. In fact, we can safely assert that the epidemic has passed the exponential phase in some states in the USA and in Canada and Australia. However, for some European countries there seems to be no compulsive reason yet to postulate a departure from the exponential law for the spread of the virus (this statement refers to the situation in 1987).

2. A simple model: Fictopia

For the exact mathematical analysis of the transients the reader can consult Gonzalez and Koch (1986). Nevertheless, the essential mathematical ideas are easy and can be explained by means of a simplified model which contains the main traits. We look at the epidemic of the freely invented fatal syndrome (FIFS) in Fictopia. This syndrome is caused by the fatality-associated virus (FAV), and initally spreads according to a pure exponential law for the cumulative number of virus carriers with a constant doubling time of 1 year. Every virus carrier develops FIFS with the probability distribution for the incubation period shown as the histogram in Fig. 10.1.

A very simple computation gives the (average) cumulative number of FIFS patients (Table 10.1). For this it is convenient to imagine that the length of the incubation period is a property of the infected subject, i.e. every virus carrier belongs to a specific incubation class 1, 2, 3, 4, or 5, where the number specifies how many years the incubation lasts. In agreement with the incubation period distribution 10 per cent belongs to incubation class 1. Accordingly, the series 10, 10, 20, 40, 80, . . . of new virus carriers appearing at year 0, 1, 2, 3, 4, . . . leads to an epidemic of FIFS cases among the class 1 virus carriers beginning at year 1 which displays the same exponential pattern as the curve of FAV carriers itself: 1, 1, 2, 4, 8, . . . (Table 10.1, column 5). Similarly, since 20 per cent of the FAV carriers belong to class 2 we obtain another exponential epidemic of FIFS cases beginning 1 year later (at year 2): 2, 2, 4, 8, 16, . . . (Table 10.1, column 6). Again, at years 3, 4, and 5 new exponential epidemics of FIFS begin for class 3, 4, and 5 FAV carriers (Table 10.1, columns 7–9). However, the health authorities in Fictopia cannot recognize the incubation class of the FIFS cases as they appear. All they see is

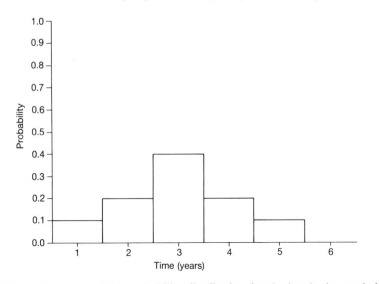

Fig. 10.1.   Histogram of the probability distribution for the incubation period of FIFS in Fictopia.

the aggregate number of FIFS cases as recorded in Table 10.1. As column 12 of Table 10.1 shows, the observable FIFS epidemic initially grows at an alarming rate (it doubles every 6 months). However, Fictopians feel reassured by the marked slowing down of the FIFS epidemic: 5 years later the doubling time has already increased by 100 per cent to 12 months, and everybody expects this trend to continue. Since the spread of the FAV is invisible, they are not aware that the number of virus carriers is doubling every 12 months (Table 10.1, column 4) nor do they recognize that the increase in the doubling time at the onset of the FIFS epidemic is a *transient*: . . . [a] temporary phenomenon occurring in a system prior to reaching a steady-state condition (*McGraw-Hill Dictionary of Scientific and Technical Terms*, 1976). The mechanism of the onset transient is clearly displayed in columns 5–9: a delayed superposition of individual epidemics, each of exponential character, boosts the aggregate FIFS epidemic. This effect passes when all incubation classes contribute to the epidemic.

It is important to view the onset transient from a different point of view: the very fact that the epidemic starts with a transitory phase having doubling times which are shorter than those of the background spread of the FAV means that we are dealing with 'anticipated' cases. This effect of anticipation can be measured by comparison with the number of FIFS cases that there would be if the epidemic were growing at the same rate as the background virus was spreading, i.e. with doubling time of 12 months. At year 2 this would give two cases while in reality there are four FIFS patients (100 per

Table 10.1. FIFS epidemic in Fictopia (first case, with constant growth rate for infections).

Time (years)	FAV carriers New	FAV carriers Cum.	Doubling time of FAV carriers (months)	Incubation type 1	2	3	4	5	FIFS cases New	FIFS cases Cum.	Doubling time of FIFS cases (months)	Anticipation effect (per cent)	A†
0	10	10	12										0.05
1	10	20	12	1					1	1		0	0.10
2	20	40	12	1	2				3	4	6.0	100	0.15
3	40	80	12	2	2	4			8	12	7.6	200	0.16
4	80	160	12	4	4	4	2		14	26	10.8	225	0.17
5	160	320	12	8	8	8	2	1	27	53	11.7	231	0.17
6	320	640	12	16	16	16	4	1	53	106	12.0	231	0.17
7	640	1280	12	32	32	32	8	2	106	212	12.0	231	0.17
8	1280	2560	12	64	64	64	16	4	212	424	12.0	231	0.17
9	2560	5120	12	128	128	128	32	8	424	848	12.0	231	0.17

†Apparency (see text).

cent more). At year 3, with a doubling time of 12 months there would be four cases while the actual observed number is 12 (200 per cent more). The anticipation effect grows until year 5 when it achieves its steady state value of 231 per cent (Table 10.1). Again, we are dealing with a transitory phenomenon, i.e. yet another manifestation of the onset transient. (A word of caution: the anticipation effect is very sensitive to the initial condition of the number of virus carriers at year 0. For instance, if the FIFS epidemic were to start with a single virus carrier the steady state would be reached with 19 per cent of anticipated cases.)

The onset transient manifests itself in several quantities of epidemiological interest. For instance, the proportion

$$A = \frac{\text{no. of FIFS cases}}{\text{no. of FAV carriers}},$$

which we have termed the apparency of the epidemic (Gonzalez and Koch 1987), displays transient behaviour through the first 5 years of the FIFS epidemic (Table 10.1, column 14).

Fictopians are deceived by another feature of the novel FIFS epidemic. Indeed, the first FIFS case has an incubation period of 1 year. After 2 years the average incubation period is 1.5 years. Thus, the erroneous impression is created that we are dealing with a disease with an incubation period of 1–2 years. As time passes some people find that the apparent average incubation period is somewhat longer, i.e. 2.2 years by year 5. However, the genuine average incubation period (Fig. 10.1) is *3.0 years*, i.e. 36 per cent higher than the apparent incubation period for the full-blown FIFS cases. The point is that the steady growth of the number of FAV carriers leads to an over-representation of short incubation periods among the manifest FIFS cases. Notice that the increase of the apparent average incubation period from 1.0 year initially to 2.2 years later on is yet another manifestation of the onset transient (Gonzalez and Koch 1987, Koch, L'age-Stehr, Gonzalez, and Dörner 1987).

The onset transient is a prototype of a positive transient (see Section 1). Negative transients arise when the spread of the virus decelerates. Because of the deceleration the statistics of the epidemic will initially contain fewer cases with very short incubation periods. Later on expected cases with short, medium, long, and very long incubation periods are missing. Altogether a subtractive or *negative* phenomenon is observed on the curve of expected cases. An illustration of how such negative transients arise is given in Section 4. It is important to realize that transients are universal phenomena associated with changes in the rate of spread of the infections which occur regardless of the actual mathematical law describing the dependence of the number of infected people on time and the specific incubation period distribution (in particular, it is irrelevant whether the incubation period distribution is symmetric, as for FIFS, or skew, as for AIDS). Of course, the actual mathematical laws for both (spreading of infection and incubation period distribution) determine the quantitative contribution of transients to the reported cases.

In the case of AIDS the average and the standard deviation of the incubation period are very long. An important study of transfusion-induced cases found an average incubation period of approximately 5 years and a standard deviation of nearly 3 years (Lawrence *et al.* 1985; Lui, Lawrence, Morgan, Peterman, Haverkos, and Bergman 1986). A more recent study of transfusion-induced cases found even longer average incubation periods of the order of 8 years (Peterman, Holmberg, and Lui 1987). There are also indications that the average incubation period for male homosexual cases may be of the order of 8 years or more (Tillett 1988). Hence transients extending for 5 years or longer occur whenever the rate of spread of the virus changes. It is not unreasonable to expect that the onset transient has 'deceived' some curve-fit analysis to yield projections which are too optimistic. A combination of a positive onset transient and one (or more) subsequent negative transient(s) due to genuine drop(s) in the rate of spread of the virus may have happened in some countries. Predictions for the AIDS epidemic should be carefully reconsidered in order to eliminate spurious effects due to transients.

3. The analysis of the AIDS epidemic in several countries

The results of the actual analysis of the total AIDS cases in the FRG, Switzerland, Austria, Australia, Canada, and the UK are presented in this section. In all cases an exponential law for the virus spread leads to good agreement with the reported cases during an initial time interval of several years through the distortion of the curve due to the onset transient. The main difference between FIFS in Fictopia and real AIDS in any country is that the incubation period for the latter has a continuous skew probability function density. This leads to a more complicated mathematical analysis which, however, is not different in essence from the one presented above. We have applied our mathematical formalism (Gonzalez and Koch 1986, 1987, 1988) to the AIDS epidemic in several countries. We take the probability density function for the incubation period (Fig. 10.2) as a gamma distribution with an average incubation period of 60 months and a standard deviation of 34 months (these values are approximately the same as those found by Lawrence *et al.* (1985) and Lui *et al.* (1986). The analysis follows similar paths in all cases. There are three essential points. First, during the initial stage the curve describing the number of virus carriers should be well approximated by an exponential curve (this point is substantiated by the agreement of our predictions with recorded cases and by comparison with the logistic curve (Gonzalez and Koch 1987). Second, when most of the onset transient has passed after 3–5 years,

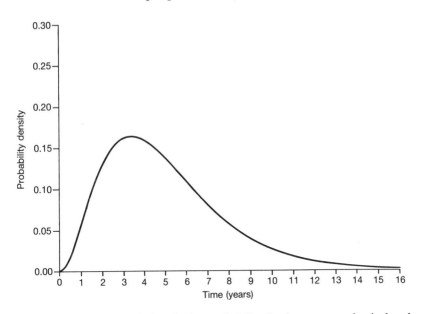

Fig. 10.2.   As a model for the incubation period distribution we use a classical probability distribution known as the gamma distribution. The average μ is 60 months and the standard deviation σ is 34 months.

the curve for AIDS cases has basically the same growth rate as that for the virus carriers (see Section 2). Finally, we assume that a constant (though unknown) proportion of virus carriers, which we shall call *fatally* infected virus carriers, develop AIDS.

We discuss Canada in detail and summarize the results for the other countries (for more details see Gonzalez and Koch 1986, 1987). It is well known that there is a considerable delay in reporting diagnosed cases to the official agencies (Curran, Meade Morgan, Hardy, Jaffe, Darrow, and Dowdle 1985; Gonzalez and Koch 1987). The numbers of diagnosed cases are definitely too low for at least the 12 months prior to the release date of the statistics. In order to keep the analysis simple we do not here discuss methods to adjust for the delay in reporting (for such methods see Downs *et al.* 1988; Heisterkamp, Jager, Downs, van Druten, and Ruitenberg 1988). Instead, we simply base our analysis on the statistics of AIDS cases by date of diagnosis between the onset of the epidemic in Canada in 1979 and the fourth quarter of 1985, i.e. we ignore the cases diagnosed during 1986 as reported to the Laboratory Centre for Disease Control, Ottawa, by 4 August 1987. Comparison with previous releases of the AIDS statistics in Canada seem to indicate that delays in reporting by more than 12 months do not have more than a marginal effect on the final data (less than 2 per cent). For Canada, a

Table 10.2. AIDS epidemic in Canada.

Time (year (quarter))	AIDS Empirical	Computed	Doubling time (months)
1979 (IV)	1	1 (1.2)	5.8
1980 (IV)	4	4 (4.4)	7.1
1981 (IV)	10	13 (13.3)	8.2
1982 (IV)	32	35 (35.5)	8.8
1983 (I)	46	45 (45.0)	8.9
1983 (II)	61	56 (56.8)	9.0
1983 (III)	71	71 (71.5)	9.1
1983 (IV)	85	89 (89.9)	9.1
1984 (I)	113	112 (112.9)	9.2
1984 (II)	146	141 (141.6)	9.2
1984 (III)	185	177 (177.4)	9.3
1984 (IV)	226	222 (222.1)	9.3
1985 (I)	284	277 (277.8)	9.3
1985 (II)	359	347 (347.3)	9.3
1985 (III)	447	434 (434.0)	9.3
1985 (IV)	540	542 (542.1)	9.4
1986 (I)	628†	676	9.4
1986 (II)	745†	845	9.4
1986 (III)	859†	1054	9.4
1986 (IV)	986†	1316	9.4

Theoretical results with average incubation period $\mu = 5.0$ years, standard deviation $\sigma = 2.8$ years, and an assumed doubling time of 9.4 months.
†Because of the delay in the reporting of the diagnosed cases these numbers must be expected to rise.

linear least-squares-fit analysis to the logarithm of the number of AIDS cases gives doubling times of roughly 6 months for the first portion of the curve of reported cases and 9.4 months for the part of the curve in 1984–1985. We interpret the last number as the doubling time *after* (most of) the onset transient has passed (of course every subpopulation, i.e. homosexuals, intravenous drug addicts, etc., has its own transient, but on account of the dominance of homosexual patients we ignore this complication for Canada). Thus we assume a pure exponential curve with a doubling time of 9.4 months for the curve describing the development of virus carriers. The results of our numerical evaluation are presented in Table 10.2. This evaluation represents our best fit obtained with an initial value of four fatal infections at the beginning of the second quarter of 1977. We expect the numbers marked with asterisks to rise because of the delay in reporting diagnosed cases. Hence, the disagreement with the computed numbers for 1986 will become less marked. It is even possible that the final figures for the diagnosed cases in 1986 could be in agreement with our simple exponential model for the spread of the virus. However, it is more likely that 1986 will mark the beginning of a departure from the exponential growth of virus carriers in Canada. The effect of the onset transient is displayed in Table 10.2, again in terms of the increase in the doubling times of the computed numbers of AIDS cases. It is seen that the effect of the transient is strongest at the beginning. As a measure of the agreement between the observed cases and predicted numbers we used the sum of fractional squares (SFS) taken over all observations. The fractional square at each observation point is defined as

$$\left(\frac{\text{predicted no.} - \text{diagnosed cases}}{\text{predicted no.}} \right)^2 .$$

By dividing the square of each discrepancy by the square of the predicted value (rather than by the first power of the predicted value as in the χ^2 case) we can deal better with curves growing from unity to several hundreds. We used the minimal value of the SFS as a criterion for the best fit. The SFS for our analysis of Canada is 0.12. For comparison, the best fit for an exponential model for the cumulative incidence of AIDS yields SFS = 0.31.

Figures 10.3 and 10.4 show results for our analysis for various countries. Notice that the data for Austria and Switzerland are still preliminary and so, therefore, is our analysis. Nevertheless, our prediction is in good agreement with the number of cases observed after our analysis had been carried out.

A byproduct of our analysis is the apparency (Gonzalez and Koch 1987, 1988).

$$A = \frac{\text{no. of AIDS cases}}{\text{no. of fatally infected people}} .$$

Remember that we assume that a constant, though unknown, fraction of virus carriers—the fatally infected carriers—develop AIDS. As a manifestation of the onset transient the apparency increases in an analogous manner to the doubling time from 2.8 to 6.4 per cent for Canada, and similarly for other countries. It is generally believed that the ratio of AIDS cases to HIV carriers is of the order of 1 per cent or less (Koch 1987). If this is correct, the ratio F of fatally infected carriers to virus carriers (the *fatality*) (Gonzalez and Koch 1987, 1988) must be of the order of 1/5, meaning that a proportion of roughly 20 per cent of the infected persons will develop AIDS (in the sense of CDC) sooner or later. Such a proportion would have seemed very pessimistic a few years ago, but today it has to be considered as much too optimistic. Several workers (Seale 1985; Koch 1985, 1987) have argued that the close kinship between HIV and other lentiviruses has ominous implications. For

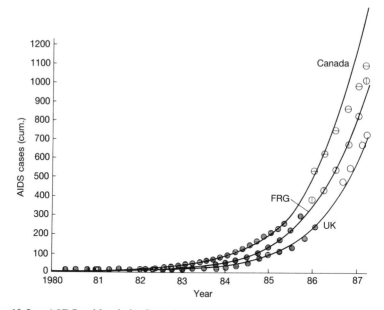

Fig. 10.3. AIDS epidemic in Canada, the FRG, and the UK. The solid curves are our predictions. The observed cases recorded before and after our analysis was carried out are indicated. Our analysis is based on an exponential curve for virus carriers with doubling times of 9.4 months (Canada), 8.8 months (FRG) and 9.3 months (UK).

instance, penetrance (and mortality) for sheep infected by visna-maedi virus is up to 100 per cent (Pálsson 1976). If the AIDS virus is comparable with its cousin in this respect, the fatality F ought to be several times (two to five times) higher than our estimate. A repetition of the analysis presented above using such hypothetical values of F leads to average incubation periods of the order of 7–12 years. We know from ongoing studies (Mathur-Wagh and coworkers, New York, and Brodt and coworkers, Frankfurt) that the progression rate to AIDS seems to peak at more than 10 per cent per year, which is consistent with many other observations (Koch 1985, 1987). A long follow-up has shown a 49 per cent progression to AIDS within 6 years, i.e. an average of 8 per cent per year (Mathur-Wagh *et al.* 1984; Mathur-Wagh, Mildwan, and Senie 1985; Mathur-Wagh 1987). A recent German study (Brodt *et al.* 1986; Helm 1987) confirms this tendency and leaves little hope that HIV carriers will not progress to AIDS or other fatal manifestations. All this indicates that the mean incubation period for general AIDS cases might well be considerable longer than inferred in the first study of transfusion-induced cases (Lawrence *et al.* 1985; Lui *et al.* 1986). Indeed, a recent update leads to significantly longer incubation periods (Peterman *et al.* 1987). Data for sexually transmitted HIV infection in male homosexuals seem to confirm this (Tillett 1988). For comparison we have carried out computations for the AIDS epidemic in Canada with an incubation period distribution (a gamma distribution) with an average period μ of 10 years and a standard deviation σ of 6 years. The predicted AIDS cases do not differ substantially from our results presented above during the initial phase of the epidemic (Gonzalez and Koch 1987). In the first years of the AIDS epidemic it is the initial part of the incubation period distribution which mainly determines the course of events. At this stage the prognostic analysis is quite insensitive to the tail of the incubation period distribution. In other words the good agreement between our prognosis and the observed numbers of AIDS cases only confirms that the incubation period distribution obtained from transfusion-induced cases (Lawrence *et al.* 1985; Lui *et al.* 1986) is a reasonably good model for short and medium-short incubation periods for the dominant risk groups, i.e. male homosexuals and intraveneous drug addicts (here we are hinting that the incubation periods for a lentivirus infection should be expected to depend on the infection modus and the typical infection dosis). The possible underestimation of the long tail of the incubation period distribution only shows up in that the values given for the number of incubating people are too low, i.e. the values of the apparency A become too small.

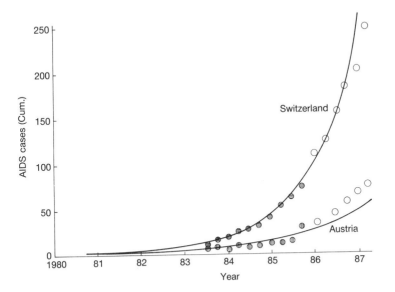

Fig. 10.4. AIDS epidemic in Switzerland and Austria. The full curves are our predictions. The observed cases recorded before and after our analysis was carried out are indicated. Our analysis is based on an exponential curve for virus carriers with doubling times of 9.9 months (Switzerland) and 15.6 months (Austria).

Table 10.3. FIFS epidemic in Fictopia (second case, with stop of infections).

Time (years)	Virus carriers		FIFS (cumulated)	Doubling time (months)
	New	Cumulated		
0	10	10	0	
1	10	20	1	
2	20	40	4	6.0
3	40	80	12	7.6
4	80	160	26	10.8
5	160	320	53	11.7
6	320	640	106	12.0
7	0	640	212	12.0
8	0	640	360	15.7
9	0	640	528	21.7
10	0	640	608	59.0
11	0	640	640	162.2
12	0	640	640	∞

4. Slow-down of the epidemic

Inhibitory factors can be roughly classified in three groups: saturation effects, in the sense that transmission of the virus to people who are already infected does not augment the size of the epidemic, prophylactic measures (such as 'safe-sex' propagation for male homosexuals and bisexuals, screening for antibodies in blood donors, etc.), and spontaneous changes in behaviour. When the growth rate of the epidemic in a given compartment decays, new types of transient effects appear in the curve of the AIDS epidemic. These will be seen very often in many forms in practically all compartments. Such effects are already occurring in early 'starters' like New York City and San Francisco, and in several states in the USA.

A qualitative illustration of the mechanism can be given by means of two examples. First, let us assume that in a compartment in Fictopia the spread of infections stops at year 6 with 64 infected people (Table 10.3). It can be seen from Table 10.3, column 5, that the FIFS epidemic slows down to zero growth over a period of 5 years. Second, let us suppose that in another compartment the growth rate for infections suddenly drops to 50 per cent, which means that the doubling time for the spread of infections is 20.5 months at year 7 (Table 10.4). The actual FIFS epidemic does not achieve the same asymptotic growth rate of 50 per cent until year 13, but the decay is anticipated through a transient starting at year 8 (Table 10.4, column 5).

Table 10.4. FIFS epidemic in Fictopia (third case, with onset of reduced growth).

Time (years)	Virus carriers		FIFS (cumulated)	Doubling time (months)
	New	Cumulated		
0	10	10	0	
1	10	20	1	
2	20	40	4	6.0
3	40	80	12	7.6
4	80	160	26	10.8
5	160	320	53	11.7
6	320	640	106	12.0
7	320	960	212	12.0
8	480	1440	392	13.5
9	720	2160	672	15.4
10	1080	3240	1048	18.7
11	1620	4860	1582	20.2
12	2430	7290	2382	20.3
13	3640	10930	3573	20.5
14	5470	16400	5359	20.5

In the final part of this section we deal with the first type of inhibitory factor (saturation effects) in the AIDS epidemic. Our main concern is to illustrate how transients influence important epidemiological properties. In previous papers we have used the same approach to obtain estimates for the time when the exponential phase should go over to less pronounced growth in different countries, i.e. for when the initial phase of the epidemic should pass (Gonzalez and Koch 1986, 1987, 1988). Modelling the total effect of the inhibitory factors has been studied by van Druten, de Boo, Jager, Heisterkamp, Coutinho, and Ruitenberg (1986) and van Druten *et al.* (1988).

Once the initial stage of the epidemic is over, the number of virus carriers is no longer small compared with the total number of susceptibles, i.e. the first condition characterizing the initial phase of the epidemic does not hold (see Section 1). We assume that the second condition defining the initial stage—equality of factors governing the infectious contacts—is still valid. Assuming in addition that the rate of infection is proportional to the fraction of susceptibles, we can derive a simple mathematical equation which is well known as the logistic model (developed by Verhulst in 1838 to account for the growth of populations and later on widely used in many applications including epidemiology (Bailey 1975)). The logistic function contains three parameters. Two of them are identical with the parameters characterizing an exponentially growing function (i.e. initial value and differential rate of growth, with the last being related to the doubling time in the exponential

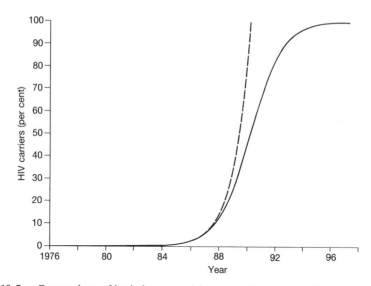

Fig. 10.5. Comparison of logistic curve with exponential function for virus carriers in high risk groups in Canada. The size of the high risk groups is assumed to be about 1.5 per cent of Canada's population. The initial parameters of the logistic function are put equal to those of the exponential curve. (Notice that the logistic curve becomes unrealistic in the asymptotic region since it predicts that all susceptibles becomes infected.)

case). The third parameter is the total number of susceptibles in the compartment.

Figure 10.5 shows the logistic curve for HIV carriers in a hypothetical compartment consisting of 360 000 people, which is a conservative estimate of the number of high risk susceptibles in Canada. The initial parameters of the logistic function are set equal to those of the exponential model for the spread of HIV in Canada (Section 3). Notice that the exponential curve for HIV carriers (broken curve) begins to differ noticeably from the logistic curve around 1987. In Section 3 we found that the predictions based on an exponential model for HIV carriers had already begun to disagree with the observed incidence of AIDS at the beginning of 1986. This should mean that all types of inhibitory effects add up to induce an earlier departure from the exponential spread of HIV. Because of the time lag induced by the incubation period distribution we would expect that such a marked departure from the exponential spread of the virus should have begun 1 or 2 years earlier, i.e. 1984–1985.

Nevertheless the logistic curve is a useful model for illustrating qualitatively how transients affect important epidemiological properties. Figures 10.6 and 10.7 display the behaviour of the doubling times and of the average

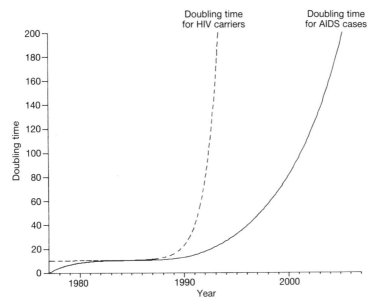

Fig. 10.6. The behaviour of the doubling times for the number of HIV carriers (broken curve) and the number of AIDS cases (solid curve). The virus spread is assumed to follow the logistic curve of Fig. 10.5. The incubation period distribution is assumed to be a gamma distribution with $\mu = 10$ years and $\sigma = 6$ years and with a cut-off of 30 years.

incubation period for the observed AIDS cases. The incubation period distribution is assumed to be a gamma distribution with average $\mu = 10$ years and standard deviation $\sigma = 6$ years. (For practical reasons, however, we assume that the longest observable incubation period is 30 years.) Figure 10.6 shows the behaviour of the doubling time for the cumulative numbers of HIV carriers and AIDS cases. The (positive) onset transient manifests itself in the initial stage of the epidemic in that the doubling time for the number of AIDS cases catches up with the (constant) doubling time of HIV carriers. Later, the doubling time of HIV carriers increases as a consequence of the depletion of susceptibles. The doubling time for the number of AIDS cases behaves similarly after a time lag of several years. The 'gap' that appears between the doubling times for HIV carriers and AIDS cases is a manifestation of a negative transient. We call this transient 'negative' because the slowing down of the virus spread is first seen in that cases with very short incubation periods occur less often (or are absent). Figure 10.7 shows the behaviour of the observed average incubation period for the total AIDS cases (solid curve) and for the new cases (broken curve). The (positive) onset transient is associated with a transition from extremely short incubation periods to a

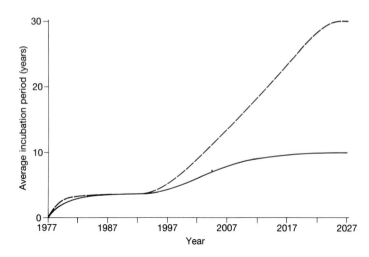

Fig. 10.7.   The behaviour of the average incubation period for the total observed AIDS cases (solid curve) and for the new AIDS cases (broken curve). The virus spread is assumed to follow the logistic curve of Fig. 10.5. The incubation period distribution is assumed to be gamma distribution with μ = 10 years and σ = 5 years and with a cut-off of 30 years.

steady state containing cases with short and long incubation periods. Notice that the average incubation period for the observed AIDS patients (solid curve) is always less than the genuine average incubation period of 10 years. Indeed, in a growing epidemic there is always an over-representation of short incubation periods. With the onset of saturation effects, cases with short incubation times soon occur less frequently, which means that the average incubation period goes up. In the final stages of the epidemic, when nearly all susceptibles are infected, the growth rate of the epidemic again decreases abruptly (see Fig. 10.5). As a consequence of the marked slowing down of the virus spread the average incubation period for the observed AIDS cases again reflects the disappearance of cases with relatively short incubation periods (Fig. 10.7). At the end of the epidemic the average incubation period for the total observed AIDS cases approaches the genuine average of the incubation period distribution (10 years). The average incubation period of new cases continues to increase until the cut-off value of 30 years is reached.

   Recent work has shown that the seroconversion latency for sexually transmitted HIV can be very long (Ranki *et al.* 1987). Obviously, the observed average seroconversion latency and the seroconversion latency distribution are influenced by transients in a manner similar to the incubation period. The observed seroconversion latencies are likely to be biased towards the short side of the distribution.

   As a final comment, we mention that the apparency of the epidemic is also a sensitive indicator of transients associated with marked changes in the growth rate of the virus spread (Gonzalez and Koch 1987).

5. A simulation model for the AIDS epidemic

There are two main reasons for developing a simulation model for the AIDS epidemic. First, it can be seen that an increasing number of compartments will contribute to the epidemic and therefore its course in the future will be determined by very complex laws. Any mathematical model attempting to describe the characteristics of several compartments (i.e. their population, age distribution, relevant behaviour related to the spread of the epidemic including interaction with other compartments, etc.) necessarily leads to very complicated equations which cannot be solved exactly but which can be simulated on a computer. Second, a simulation model enables the influence of various choices of prophylactic and political actions upon the course of events to be developed.

Systems dynamics has shown us that simulation models need not to be very faithful to yield a *qualitatively* correct picture of the situation, provided that the key components and their interactions are approximately represented in the model. Hence valuable information about the feasibility, inter-dependences, and appropriate sequence of measures can be obtained even with a small simulation model. This is the present status of our model, which has been mainly developed at the University of Bamberg. We plan to improve it by incorporating more details and by refining the relations among the model parameters in accordance with increasing knowledge about real epidemics.

A detailed description of the model and the results obtained so far have been given elsewhere (Dörner 1986a,b; Koch *et al.* 1987). Here, it is sufficient to state that at present the model provides a rough frame for a city of two million inhabitants with the following compartments: prostitutes, homosexual and bisexual males, intravenous drug addicts, children (age less than 15), young people (15–25 years), middle-aged people, and old people. Every such compartment is characterized by its total population, migrations to and from other compartments, regular sexual contact with other members of the same compartment, occasional sexual contacts with members of foreign compartments, promiscuity rates, death rates (and birth rates for children), other risk factors (e.g. blood transfusions), etc. The model contains infection rates which depend on risky behaviour and on risk factors. Infected people can develop AIDS according to a probability distribution law for the incubation period, and AIDS patients may die as described by a mortality distribution.

So far we have studied the course of the epidemic by running the following trials.

(i) A 'zero trial', which is an unrealistic situation where all rates of the simulation model remain unchanged, i.e. time independent. This amounts to a situation in which no prophylactic measures are taken and there is no spontaneous behaviour change. The zero trial is comparable with the role of a control group treated with a placebo in a clinical trial. Comparisons of the zero trial with trials simulating preventive measures (see below) enable us to draw conclusions about the effects of such measures.

(ii) A trial where prostitution is eliminated at a particular point early in the epidemic. As a consequence the number of new virus carriers drops suddenly and the growth of the epidemic is delayed for about 7 years. This trial emphasizes the role of prostitution as a link between different compartments (e.g. intravenous drug addicts and the general heterosexual population).

(iii) A trial where preventive measures have the following impact early in the epidemic: (a) the infection rate for male homosexuals drops to 50 per cent of its initial value; (b) the promiscuity of the heterosexual population is reduced by 50 per cent; (c) the probability of infection in contacts with prostitutes decreases to 20 per cent of its initial value; (d) the elimination of the HIV in all types of blood product succeeds in 95 per cent of cases. As a consequence the growth of the epidemic is strongly suppressed throughout the period simulated in this trial, and this reduction is particularly conspicuous for the male homosexual population.

(iv) Other trials indicate that the reduction of promiscuity has the strongest suppressive effect upon the epidemic. Furthermore, contact between different compartments is of particular importance for the development of the epidemic. Overall, the system is dominated by a few crucial parameters. For instance a slight increase in the parameter reflecting the drug consumption and promiscuous behaviour of young people has catastrophic consequences. It is extremely important to investigate the influence and properties of these parameters in detail. If a thorough analysis confirms their dominant role it will be imperative to plan all prophylactic measures in the light of this finding.

AIDS attacks mainly young people in reproductive and professionally active age groups. The impact on modern society, which already has low birth rates, an abundance of pensioners, and a public health service under great strain, is obvious. The model simulates these effects and enables their size to be estimated for various outcomes of the epidemic.

In most countries feasible measures to combat the AIDS epidemic have not been implemented immediately. Rather, even obvious actions such as screening blood products for antibodies have been delayed for months (in some countries even for years). But it is a sad fact that growth processes follow a quasi-exponential pattern. A delay in carrying out a necessary measure means that there will be additional tens of thousands of victims in later years. The simulation model bears this out and yields the order of magnitude of these effects. Pairs of trials were run to compare the effect of delaying certain measures by 1 year. For instance, screening for antibodies in blood products and measures to reduce the infection probabilities were introduced either 3 or 4 years after the onset of the epidemic. The consequence of delaying these prophylactic actions was that 14 years later an additional 13 000 AIDS deaths occurred. In combatting AIDS there is very little time to spare. Everybody in a position to influence the course of events should be aware of this.

6. Simsim programming and simulation of the AIDS epidemic

SIMSIM is a fourth-generation tool developed by two of us (MM and LV) for programming computer simulation models. It is written in simple language so that people who possess the relevant knowledge of the system to be modelled are able to develop a computer simulation model without having to engage computer specialists. It provides a powerful system for writing, testing, running, and modifying computer simulation models and for choosing the appropriate presentation of the results. The programming tool, SIMTEK, is menu oriented and contains a screen-oriented editor, a proof-reader to check the syntax of the program, an interpreter to carry out and present the results in tabular or graphic form, and a translator to generate code in general-purpose programming languages such as Pascal or C. At present SIMSIM is available for the IBM PC and compatible machines, as well as for the SCANDIS/COMPIS microcomputer. Three of us (JJG, MM, and LV) are participating in a project sponsored by the Norwegian Datasekretariatet, which operates under the auspices of the Ministry of Education, to develop simulation models of the AIDS epidemic for use at Norwegian secondary schools.

References

Bailey, N.T.J. (1975). *The mathematical theory of infectious diseases and its applications*. Hafner, New York.

Barré-Sinoussi, F., Chermann, J.C., Rey, F., Nugeyre, M.T., ChaMaret, S., Gruet, J., Dauguet, C., Axler-Blin, C., Vézinet-Brun, F., Rouzioux, C., Rozenbaum, W., and Montagnier, L. (1983). Isolation of a T-lymphotrophic retrovirus from a patient at risk for AIDS. *Science* **220**, 868–71.

Brodt, H.R., Helm, E.B., Werner, A., Jötten, A., Bergmann, L., Küver, A., and Stille, W. (1986). Verlaufsbeobachtungen bei Personen sus AIDS-Risikogruppen bzw. mit LAV/HTLV III Infektion. *Deutsche Medizinische Wochenschrift* **31/32** 1175–80.

Curran, J.W., Meade Morgan, W., Hardy, A.M., Jaffe, H.W., Darrow, W.W., and Dowdle, W.R. (1985). The epidemiology of AIDS: current status and future prospects. *Science* **229**, 1352–7.

Dörner, D. (1986a). Ein Simulationsprogram für die Ausbreitung von AIDS. *Memorandum 40, Projekt Systemdenken*. Universität Bamberg.

Dörner, D. (1986b). Addendum zum Memorandum 40. *Memorandum 40 Add, Projekt Systemdenken*. Universität Bamberg.

Downs, A.M., Ancelle, R.A., Jager, J.C., and Brunet, J.B. (1987). AIDS in Europe: current trends and short-term predictions estimated from surveillance data. *AIDS* 1, 53-7.

Downs, A.M., Ancelle, R. Jager, J.C., Heisterkamp, S.H., van Druten, J.A.M., Ruitenberg, E.J., and Brunet, J.B. (1988). The statistical estimation, from routine surveillance data, of past, present, and future trends in AIDS incidence in Europe. These *Proceedings*, pp. 1-16.

van Druten, J.A.M., de Boo, Th. Jager, J.C., Heisterkamp, S.H., Coutinho, R.A., and Ruitenberg, E.J. (1986). AIDS prediction and intervention. Lancet i, 852-3.

van Druten, J.A.M., de Boo, Th., Reintjes, A.G.M., Jager, J.C., Heisterkamp, S.H., Coutinho, R.A., Bos, J.M., and Ruitenberg, E.J. (1988). Reconstruction and prediction of spread of HIV infection in populations of homosexual men. These *Proceedings*, pp. 52-76.

González, J.J. and Koch, M.G. (1986). On the role of transients for the prognostic analysis of AIDS and the anciennity distribution of AIDS patients. *AIDS-Forschung (AIFO)* 11, 621-30.

González, J.J. and Koch, M.G. (1988). The prognostic analysis of AIDS: incubation period, transients, and anciennity distribution (in Italian). In: *AIDS. Diagnosi, prevenzione, terapia. Proceedings of the 1st International Meeting of AVIS on AIDS, Naples, 6-8 December 1985*. Solei, Milan pp. 255-307.

González, J.J. and Koch, M.G. (1987). On the role of 'transients' (biasing transitional effects) for the prognostic analysis of the AIDS epidemic. *American Journal of Epidemiology* 126, 985-1005.

Heisterkamp, S.H., Jager, J.C., Downs, A.M., van Druten, J.A.M., and Ruitenberg, E.J. (1988). Statistical estimation of AIDS incidence from surveillance data and the link with modelling of trends. These *Proceedings*, pp. 17-25.

Helm, E.B. (1987). Personal communication.

Karpas, A. (1983). Unusual virus produced by cultured cells from a patient with AIDS. *Molecular Biology and Medicine* 1, 457-9.

Koch, M.G. (1985). *AIDS—vår framtid?* Svenska Carnegie Institutet, Stockholm.

Koch, M.G. (1987). *AIDS—vom Molekül zur Pandemie*. Spektrum, Heidelberg.

Koch, M.G., L'age-Stehr, J.González, J.J., Dörner, D. (1987). Die Epidemiologie von AIDS. *Spektrum der Wissenschaft* 8, 38-51.

Lawrence, D.N., Lui, K.J., Bregman, D.J. *et al.* (1985). A model-based estimate of the average incubation and latency period for transfusion-associated AIDS. *Abstracts of the International Conference on AIDS, Atlanta, GA, April 14-17 1985*.

Levy, J.A., Hoffman, A.D., Kramer, S.M., Peterman, T.A., and Morgan, W.M. (1984). Isolation of lymphocytopathic retroviruses from San Francisco patients with AIDS. *Science* 225, 840-2.

Lui, K.J., Lawrence, D.N., Morgan, W.M., Peterman, T.A., Haverkos, H.W., and Bregman, D.J. (1986). A model-based approach to estimating the mean incubation period for transfusion-associated acquired immunodeficiency syndrome. *Proceedings of the National Academy of Sciences of the USA* 83, 305-5.

McGraw-Hill dictionary of scientific and technical terms (1976). McGraw-Hill, New York.

Mathur-Wagh, U. (1987). Personal communication.

Mathur-Wagh, U., Enlow, R.W., Spigland, I. *et al.* (1984). Longitudinal study of persistent generalized lymphadenopathy in homosexual men: relation to AIDS. *Lancet* **i**, 1033–8.

Mathur-Wagh, U., Mildwan, D. and Senie, R.T. (1985). Follow-up at 4.5 years on homosexual men with generalized lymphadenopathy. *New England Journal of Medicine* **313**, 1542–3.

Pálsson, P.A. (1976). Maedi and visna in sheep. In *Slow virus diseases of animals and man* (ed. R.M. Kimberlin). North-Holland, Amsterdam.

Peterman, T.A., Holmberg, S.D., and Lui, K.J. (1987). Transfusion-associated AIDS in the United States. *Abstracts of the 3rd International Conference on AIDS, Washington, DC, J1–5 June 1987*, p. 160.

Popovic, M., Sarngadharan, M.G., Read, E., *et al.* (1984). Detection, isolation, and continuous production of cytopathic retroviruses, (HTLV III) from patients with AIDS and pre-AIDS. *Science* **224**, 497–500.

Ranki, A., Valle, S.L., Krohn, M., Antonen, J., Allain, J.P., Leuther, M., Franchini, G. and Krohn, K. (1987). Long latency precedes overt seroconversion in sexually transmitted HIV infection. *Lancet* **ii**, 589–93.

Seale, J. (1985). AIDS virus infection: prognosis and transmission. *Journal of the Royal Society of Medicine* **78**, 613–15.

Tillett, H.E. (1988). Observations from the UK epidemic. These *Proceedings*, pp. 26–9.

Tillett, H.E. and McEvoy, M. (1986). Reassessment of predicted numbers of AIDS cases in the UK. *Lancet* **ii**, 1104.

11

Computer simulations of the AIDS epidemic in the Federal Republic of Germany

S. Stannat, D. Kiessling, I. Schedel, and H. Deicher

1. Introduction

Because of the fragmentary nature of epidemiological data and the variations in the behaviour of particular groups in the population alternative mathematical models for the spread of HIV infection are required. Our approach to the problem was to analyse known data, to define the essential parameters for a suitable model, and to compensate for the paucity of data by using the results of rough calculations and retrospective computer runs (Kiessling, Stannat, Schedel, and Deicher 1986).

2. Model assumptions

We concentrated on sexual intercourse as it is the epidemiologically most relevant mode of virus transmission. In the FRG the sexually active part of the population (40 million people) was divided into six groups exhibiting different sexual behaviour according to data from surveys (Dannecker and Reiche 1974; Habermehl and Eichner 1978) (Fig. 11.1). Four per cent of the male population were assumed to be active homosexuals, and they were subdivided into one group with lower promiscuity (HOM1) and a smaller group with higher promiscuity (HOM2). In addition, 2 per cent of the male population were assumed to be bisexually active (BIS). It is hard to give an exact definition which covers all types of female prostitution and to define the number of prostitutes, but for this model we assumed a value of 0.1 per cent of the total population (Höpken 1986).

For the following reasons and without any evident loss of statistical accuracy, we ignored the birth rate and the natural death rate:

the mortality rate of uninfected persons and compensation by seronegative adolescents entering the sexually active age group does not affect the epidemiological situation;
there would be a need not only for the applied 'average' but also for age-specific epidemiological data which are far beyond the bounds of current knowledge;

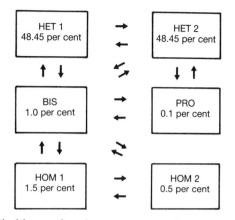

Fig. 11.1. Statistical interactions between groups of the population with different sexual behaviour (percentage of total sexually active population): HET1, heterosexuals with 'low' promiscuity; HET2, heterosexuals with 'high' promiscuity; BIS, bisexually active men; PRO, female prostitutes; HOM1, homosexually active men with 'low' promiscuity; HOM2, homosexually active men with 'high' promiscuity.

because of the influence of possible new factors on the infectiological situation (e.g. changes in sexual behaviour or the introduction of a vaccine against HIV infections), our model is not meant to be a long-term projection.

2.1 First infection

On the basis of known epidemiological data (Vogt, Bettex, and Lüthy 1983) we assumed that in January 1981 a number t_0 of 1000 HIV positives at different stages of the disease were distributed in the ratio 700:200:100 among the three homosexually active groups HOM2, HOM1, and BIS. A doubling time of 12 months was assumed, and the statistical dates of virus acquisition were estimated by applying a decreasing exponential function into the past.

2.2 Interactions

To assist with the mathematical processing of interactions among the population we introduced the term 'acquisition of a new sexual contact' (ac). This implies not only a single new contact but the sum of *all sexual contacts within a new partnership*. Thus further applications of uncertain data—such as the number of sexual contacts and different sexual practices taking place within one partnership, the introduction of a special 'risk factor' for each practice, etc.—are avoided by using average values. No further distinction between males and females was made.

The male homosexuals of the subgroup HOM1 (n_{HOM1} = 600 000) are assumed to have an average of c_{HOM1} = 10 different homosexual partners per year; the more sexually active subgroup HOM2 consists of n_{HOM2} = 200 000 male homosexuals with an average of c_{HOM2} = 50 different homosexual partners per year (according to the distribution of partners reported by Dannecker and Reiche 1974, and Habermehl and Eichner 1978). Therefore HOM1 'offers' 6 000 000 new homosexual contacts per year which remain at random within HOM1 or are directed to HOM2 and BIS. The total number of 'acquired new sexual contacts' within the homosexual subgroups (ac_{HOM}) is calculated as follows:

$$ac_{HOM} = n_{HOM1} c_{HOM1} + n_{HOM2} c_{HOM2} + n_{BIS} c_{BIS}.$$

The distribution probability for any homosexual contact to be directed to the HOM1 subgroup is

$$q_{HOM1} = \frac{n_{HOM1} c_{HOM1}}{ac_{HOM}}$$

analogously

$$q_{HOM2} = \frac{n_{HOM2} c_{HOM2}}{ac_{HOM}}$$

to be directed to HOM2. Interactions between the other groups are calculated similarly (the exact equations are given by Kiessling *et al.* 1986).

The probability of HIV infection after 'acquisition of a new sexual contact' is determined by the contagion index ci. The number N_{inf} of new infections in a non-infected group N as a result of contacts between members of that group and members of another group x in which some people are already infected is given by

$$N_{inf} = (ac)(ci) \frac{X_{inf}}{X}$$

where ac is the number of new sexual contacts acquired and ci is the contagion index. N_{inf} is calculated for each interaction separately on a monthly basis. If there is contact between two infected persons, they cannot become infected twice; this is taken into account by an additional factor for statistical correction ($f_c = 1 - X_{inf}/X$). Infected people remain infectious for the rest of their lives.

2.3 Possible pathways

Figure 11.2 shows the possible pathways within this model. If an infection occurs, the initial manifestation index mi_i defines whether the person will develop manifest AIDS or only a permanent infectious state ranging from symptomless seropositivity to all AIDS-related conditions. In addition, we suggest that a certain proportion of the pool of virus carriers will con-

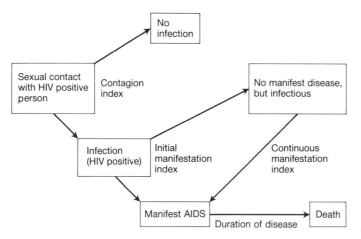

Fig. 11.2. Possible pathways after sexual contact with an HIV-positive individual.

tinuously develop the lethal manifest disease, either spontaneously or as a result of 'promoting factors' such as intercurrent infections. This continuous manifestation index mi_c corresponds to the reported very variable incubation period (the theoretical range of mi_c is discussed by Kiessling *et al.* (1986)).

2.4 Estimation of manifestation index
The (initial and/or continuous) manifestation index in the 'average' population is not exactly known. Polk *et al.* (1987) give a figure of 59 AIDS cases in a cohort of 1835 seropositive homosexual men during a medium follow-up of 15 months, i.e. approximately 2.6 per cent per year. Application of this manifestation index to the estimated number of at least 200 000 seropositive homosexual men in the FRG would give a figure of 5 200 *new* AIDS cases per year. This is far greater than the real figures, even if we accept a certain number of unreported cases. A possible explanation for this discrepancy could be that most of the epidemiological studies were carried out in high risk cohorts with an assumed high rate of promoting factors. The figures used in our simulation were defined by retrospective computer runs (the results were assessed in January 1986).

3. Results

The results of our computer simulation are in good agreement with the actual epidemiological figures (Table 11.1). Several computer runs were performed to simulate the following scenarios.

The presence of 2000 HIV-positive haemophiliacs (Hunsman *et al.* 1985)

Table 11.1. Cumulative numbers of AIDS patients and deaths†.

Date	Actual figures‡		Computer simulation	
	AIDS cases	Deaths	AIDS cases	Deaths
9/1983	40	11	47	17
9/1984	100	38	122	48
9/1985	272	111	293	122
9/1986	604	293	554	294
9/1987	1400	627	1 302	654
12/1987	1669	724	1 514	784
9/1988			2 292	1 302
9/1995			16 321	13 760
9/2000			30 947	27 806

†mi_i = 0.1 per cent; mi_c = 0.25 per cent per year.
‡Taken from monthly reports of the Federal Health Office in *Bundesgesundheitsblatt*.

within the heterosexual population: no significant effect on the spread of HIV infections and AIDS cases in the population as a whole was noted.

No transmission by prostitutes: both the number of infections and the number of AIDS cases in the heterosexual groups, HET2 in particular, might be greatly reduced, since prostitutes can no longer act as 'vectors' for the virus in these groups.

Changes in sexual behaviour, e.g. by reduction of homosexual contact rates (Clumeck, van de Perre, Carael, Rouvroy, and Nzaramba 1985) to one sixth for subgroup BIS, one half for HOM1, and one fifth for HOM2 or by qualitative changes such as the use of safe-sex practices: this leads to a significantly lower increase (five times less) in AIDS cases not only in homosexuals but also in the heterosexual groups.

4. Conclusion

It is rather difficult to find a suitable mathematical model for the simulation of the dynamics of spread of HIV infections at this stage of epidemiological knowledge and virus research. In view of these uncertainties, we conclude that it is possible to use the data now available and to compensate for the present paucity of data to some extent. This model can be used to predict HIV infections, AIDS cases, and death rates expected in the next few years. These are not meant to be accurate forecasts but an approximation of possible developments. The model can be used to demonstrate the epidemiological effects of changes in sexual behaviour and their influence on the spread of HIV infections. Health politicians may find this helpful for further decisions, particularly regarding the necessity of information campaigns about safe-sex methods etc. As our understanding of the disease increases, simulation models and predictions are likely to become more accurate and reliable.

References

Clumeck, N., van de Perre, P., Carael, M., Rouvroy, D., and Nzaramba, D. (1985). Heterosexual promiscuity among African patients with AIDS. *New England Journal of Medicine* **313**, 182.

Dannecker, M. and Reiche, R. (1974). *Der gewöhnliche Homosexuelle.* Fischer-Verlag, Stuttgart.

Habermehl, W. and Eichner, K. (1978). *RALF-Report: Das Sexualverhalten der Deutschen.* Hoffmann und Campe, Hamburg.

Höpken, W. (1986). Personal communication, Public Health Office, Hannover.

Hunsman, G., Schneider, J., Bayer, H., Kurth, R., Werner, A., Brede, H.D., Erfle, V., Mellert, W., Brodt, H.R., Bergmann, L., Helm, I., Scharrer, I., Kreuz, W., Berthold, H., Wernet, P., Schneider, E.M., Schimpf, K., Egli, U., Bienzle, U., Schmitz, H., Kern, P., Krüger, G., Rasokat, H., Lechler, E., Seifried, E., Hellstern, P., Schneider, W., Holzer, E., Goebel, F.D., and Hehlmann, R. (1985). Seroepidemiology of HTLV-III (LAV) in the Federal Republic of Germany. *Klinische Wochenschrift* **63**, 233–5.

Kiessling, D., Stannat, S., Schedel, I., and Deicher, H. (1986). Überlegungen und Hochrechnungen zur Epidemiologie des 'Acquired Immunodeficiency Syndrome' in der Bundesrepublik Deutschland. *Infection* **14** 217–22.

Polk, B.F., Fox, R., Brookmeyer, R., Kanchanara, A.S., Kaslow, R., Visscher, B., Rinaldo, C., and Phair, J. (1987). Predictors of the acquired immunodeficiency syndrome developing in a cohort of seropositive homosexual men. *New England Journal of Medicine* **316**, 61–6.

Vogt, M., Bettex, J.D., and Lüthy R. (1983). Erworbenes Immundefektsyndrom (AIDS). Eine Übersicht nach zwei Jahren. *Deutsche Medizinische Wochenschrift* **50**, 1927–33.

12

Economic aspects of care and prevention of HIV infection and AIDS

A.M. Johnson

1. Introduction

The epidemic of AIDS and HIV presents a series of clinical and public health problems which have attendant economic implications. The direct costs of management of the HIV epidemic will vary considerably between one country and another. This will depend on the epidemic pattern and the future number of AIDS cases, the organization and funding of health and social services, and the success of preventive strategies to reduce the future social and financial burden of AIDS.

The cost of clinical services is likely to fall most heavily on major cities and on particular centres, at least at the start of the epidemic. For example, over 75 per cent of cases in the UK have been reported from the four Health Regions around London, and the majority of cases are managed in three inner London hospitals. In the USA disproportionate requirements for care have fallen on health services in cities such as San Francisco and New York.

In addition to clinical services for HIV-infected patients, costs arise from providing individual counselling and information programmes for members of high risk groups, from providing appropriate protection from infection for health care staff, from screening and heat treatment of blood and blood products, and from mounting public health education programmes outside the health services. Studies of the cost of care and health service use are essential, linked with appropriate epidemiological data and estimates of future AIDS cases, for any health care planning to take place. Studies of different patterns of health care use may help decision makers in planning the most efficient and effective strategies for care.

2. Direct costs of treatment for patients

Studies of direct costs of care have largely focused on the hospital care of AIDS patients. Very little has been written about costs of patients with less severe manifestations of HIV infection. Cost studies have all emphasized the considerable individual variation in requirements for care. Patients may require several hospital admissions as well as considerable psychosocial support over the course of their illness. Studies to date have shown wide variations in estimates of cost, partly because of different methodologies but also because of differences in health care organization.

Hardy, Rauch, Echenberg, Morgan, and Curran[1] estimated a lifetime cost of $147 000 per AIDS case based on an assumption of 168 hospital in-patient days per case. This figure is now generally regarded as high, reflecting the high estimates of length of stay used in their calculations. More recent studies have given lower estimates. Scitovsky, Cline, and Lee[2] estimated a mean lifetime cost per case of $27 571 for patients who had received all their care in San Francisco General Hospital and died during 1984. The mean length of stay was only 11.7 days per admission and patients spent on average of 34.7 days in hospital over a 'lifetime'. Seage *et al.*[3] estimated a lifetime cost of $50 380 for patients treated in Massachussets with total lifetime requirements for hospital care of 67 in-patient days. Their calculations were derived from observing prevalent patients over 1 year, rather than following incident cases through to death. Our own study based on cases followed to death in London estimated an average length of stay of 17.2 days per admission and 50 days per lifetime. Lifetime hospital in-patient and out-patient cost was estimated at £6,800 ($10 132) based on management on a general medical ward in a National Health Service (NHS) Teaching Hospital.[4] The studies by Scitovsky *et al.* and ourselves both emphasized that basing calculations on those who die tends disproportionately to select those with short survival time. However, it cannot be assumed that costs of care rise in proportion to survival times. Requirements for care vary according to the stage of illness and the diagnostic category. Those with Kaposi's sarcoma having lower in-patient costs over a defined time period but in turn have longer survival times.[2,5] It has also been suggested that drug users have higher requirements for in-patient care than homosexuals, owing to other medical problems associated with drug use, which may partially explain cost differences between different cities.[6]

Costing studies have all shown that over 80 per cent of hospital costs relate to in-patient care and much of this to room charges. Length of stay is therefore an important determinant of overall hospital cost, and reducing length of stay by developing community care or out-patient-based care may on balance reduce cost. Use of intensive care varies between studies and has been shown to increase cost considerably.[2,4] However, use of intensive care has now diminished in San Francisco, possibly as a result of accumulating evidence that the outcome for patients admitted to intensive care is very poor.[7] Although there are methodological differences in the costing studies discussed, as well as possible difference in the types of patient treated, the relatively short length of stay in the San Francisco study probably reflects the substantial efforts made to coordinate care, to reduce the length of stay, to develop hospice, hostel, and home care, and to depend substantially on the voluntary sector for community and social services.[2,8]

In future, changing patterns of care may alter estimates of cost per case. On the one hand development of community care may reduce cost by reducing hospital stay, but on the other hand the development of new therapies, such as azidothymidine (AZT), may, if they prolong life or are expensive themselves, increase cost.

3. Community and voluntary costs

Very little work has been done to assess the costs of community care, the costs to families or lovers, or the relative cost effectiveness of different care options such as hospital versus hospice care.

Arno[8] has documented the substantial contribution of community-based organizations to the care of AIDS patients in San Francisco. The Shanti Project, which provides community support and housing, and the Hospice Program, which provides community health care, had a total expenditure of $1 688 042 in 1984–1985. Local government provides substantial support to these groups, but private donations are the second-largest source of funding. In addition, these organizations rely substantially on donated labour. The economic value of labour donated to Hospice and Shanti alone was estimated at $838 229 in 1984–1985. In the UK we have seen a similar reliance on the voluntary sector, particularly through the Terrence Higgins Trust and gay organizations, to provide social support. Home health care has relied on existing NHS home nursing provision, and on informal caring by friends and relations. As the number of AIDS patients requiring care in London increases, there will be an increasing need for services outside hospital if pressure on acute beds is to be relieved. Schemes for privately and publicly funded hospice care are being developed.

Studies will be necessary to cost different care options. Arno[8] estimated the cost of home-based hospice care in San Francisco at $94 per day per patient, approximately 12 per cent of the cost of hospital care. However, such comparisons will in themselves depend substantially on the funding and organization of health services in different places and on the degree to which they rely on donated labour.

4. Projecting future hospital bed use

Projections of future bed use are limited not only by the uncertainties which limit predictions of future cases but also by the uncertainties which determine both current and future patterns of care. Nevertheless, they can give assistance to short-term planning and give some estimate of the potential magnitude of the impact of AIDS patients on the health care system. For the purposes of planning, it is more useful to look at prevalent rather than incident cases of AIDS and measure the number requiring hospital care at a given point in time. For example, based on data on 86 AIDS patients treated in London, we estimated that on average a patient spent approximately 1 day in hospital per week from diagnosis of AIDS. Thus, by estimating the number of AIDS patients expected to be alive at a given moment in time and assuming no change in patterns of care, we can calculate that, on average, approximately one-seventh of them will be in hospital at a given point in time. Using the revised projections by McEvoy and coworkers[5,9] for the UK and current survival rates gives an estimate of 2,338 AIDS patients alive at the end of 1988, and an estimated average bed need of 334 nationally by that time. However, the majority of these beds would be required in inner London, where hospital beds are currently being reduced. The annual cost of these beds at current cost in a London NHS Teaching Hospital would be of the order of £15.5 million ($22 640 000), representing approximately 0.08 per cent of resources consumed annually by the NHS.

Projections of bed use in the USA, based on the data of Scitovsky *et al.*[2] and estimating 145 000 cases of AIDS alive at some time during 1991, give a figure of 4.6 million bed days, which is greater then the total number of bed days occupied in the USA for lung cancer or vehicle accidents.[6,10] This amounts to 1 per cent of all hospital beds in the USA and 3 per cent of all hospital costs, with considerable geographic variation. Costs of this care, taking into account the variation in estimates of costs per case, is estimated at $8–16 billion, with the higher figure representing the worst-case scenario.

5. Costs of establishing a service

Estimates of cost per case represent only the immediate treatment costs for AIDS patients and ignore the costs of treating seropositives who have less severe manifestations of HIV infection. In the San Francisco cohort of homosexual men there were 9.4 symptomatic seropositives to manage for every case of AIDS, as well as many more asymptomatic seropositives who may be increasingly diagnosed as HIV antibody testing becomes more widely available.[11] Their need for in-patient treatment may be small, but their out-patient and counselling needs are considerable. Numerically they may add substantially to the demand for care.

It is useful to consider not only average costs but also the particular additional costs which arise from setting up services for a new disease. Marginal costs (i.e. the cost of treating one more patient within a health care system) may be relatively small when one more patient can be managed within existing resources. This cost may increase substantially if it becomes necessary to make new capital or revenue investment to manage cases. In hospitals treating few AIDS cases those patients will have relatively little effect, but in centres seeing many patients there may be considerable impact on the overall delivery of health care. In a health care system with finite resources, management of a new problem represents an opportunity cost in terms of other patients who might have been treated instead. The impact of management of AIDS and HIV infection needs to be measured and financed if a reduction in service is not to be seen elsewhere. This may require providing more hospital beds or, in the case of the NHS in London, keeping open hospital beds which might otherwise have been closed. In our study in a London Health Service District, which by 1985 had treated 18 per cent of the UK AIDS cases, we investigated the additional resources which were invested in the HIV epidemic in the financial year 1986–1987. These included a capital investment of £472 000 ($708 000) to provide a dedicated ward, to upgrade laboratories to appropriate health and safety standards, and to provide dental services for seropositives unable to obtain treatment from general dental practitioners. An additional revenue cost of £388 000 ($582 000) was estimated to run in-patient, out-patient, counselling, and laboratory services. The major revenue cost arose from the employment of new staff to take on the workload.[4]

Costs of care will in part be determined by difficult policy decisions about the management of AIDS patients. Should management be on open wards, in infectious disease units, in dedicated AIDS units, in isolation hospitals, in hospices, in hostels, or at home? How aggressive will management be, particularly in relation to intensive care units in the developed world? Such decisions will vary from one society to another and from one health care system to another, and will depend on available resources for health care. The answer to the question: 'How much does it cost to treat a case of AIDS?' will vary from Zambia to Paris, from Paris to London, and from the east coast to the west coast of the USA.

6. Who pays?

The costs of care cannot be divorced from the question of 'Who pays?' Will it be the private individual, public or private health care insurance systems, or services directly funded from central government and indirectly financed by the tax payer? Seage *et al.*[3] showed that the charge per AIDS case varied according to the source of payment. Considerable controversy has arisen in the USA over the rights of insurance companies to refuse insurance to HIV-antibody-positive individuals.[12] If they do so, it is not clear how costs of care will be met. Some may simply go without care or fall back on informal carers at home.

In the UK the additional costs of AIDS have to some extent been recognized by central government by the allocation of £3.65 million ($5.29 million) for treatment and counselling services to Health Districts in central London in 1985 and 1986. The initial 1987–1988 allocation amounted to £4.4 million ($6.38 million), again limited to the three London Regions. This sum was substantially less than the funds requested by local health authorities, and the uncertainty of future additional funding in the UK makes long-term planning fraught with financial uncertainty.[13]

7. Indirect and social costs

Infection with HIV may have a major impact on the individual and on his/her family, work, and social life. Clearly many of these 'social' costs are essentially unquantifiable in financial terms. However, attempts have been made to quantify the theoretical 'indirect' costs of lost productivity as a result of sickness and premature death. In addition, costs arise from sickness and other benefits paid to the individual. Hardy *et al.*[1] estimated that the indirect costs arising from lost productivity of the first 10 000 cases of AIDS in the USA amounted to $4.6 billion. Wells[14] estimated the indirect costs of the first 543 AIDS cases in the UK at £150 million. However, such financial valuations are conceptually open to considerable criticism, especially in a time of high unemployment. Nor does it seem acceptable to value premature loss of life in purely financial terms. It remains a stark fact that AIDS was amongst the leading causes of death in 1984 for men aged 25–54 in New York City and accounted for 24 400 years of potential life lost below the age of 65.[15,16]

8. Information and counselling for high risk groups

Counselling services for those at high risk of acquiring HIV have several purposes. They provide emotional support for those with AIDS, for those who are antibody positive, and for the worried well, whether they choose to take antibody testing or not. Such services also have an essential public health role in providing the individual with advice on how to reduce personal risk of transmitting or acquiring the virus, and are therefore an important require-ment for backing up public health education campaigns. In the USA alter-native test sites were established to provide testing and counselling, as much to prevent high risk groups seeking testing through blood donation as to prevent viral spread within high risk communities.[17] In the UK the majority of testing and counselling has taken place within sexually transmitted disease (STD) clinics. Other than in London Districts, NHS clinics have been required to fund services within existing budgets or not to provide the service.

Health Districts throughout the UK have been asked to present AIDS plans and costings. Many will request extra staff for testing and counselling and for local health education. If funds are not centrally committed in a state-financed service, choices will have to be made locally of whether services for

AIDS/HIV should take priority over others. Local areas will vary in their needs, but a conservative estimate of £50 000 per District to provide testing and counselling gives an annual cost in England and Wales of £10 million ($14.5 million).[18] Increasingly in the UK, further costs are emerging. These include the costs of setting up preventive services for drug users, which will have to include not only management and prevention of HIV infection but also drug-dependence treatment policies, and the establishment and evaluation of needle-exchange programmes.

9. Education and protection of health care staff

Included in the costs of the HIV epidemic must be an assessment of the costs of policies for controlling infection and of training staff in what does and what does not constitute a risk for infection. Such costs include such minor items as extra gloves and gowns etc. More costly requirements have arisen in the UK, for example, from adhering to health and safety guidelines for working with potentially infected specimens in the laboratory.[4,19]

10. Safety of blood and blood products

The cost of screening blood donors for HIV antibody is not inconsiderable. The cost of testing the 2.2 million units processed annually in the UK is estimated at approximately £2 million ($2.9 million). In addition, the cost of heat treatment of blood products in the UK amounts to a further £3–4 million.[13] It is interesting to reflect that in the first three million units of blood screened in the blood transfusion service in the UK 65 potentially infectious units were detected.[20] In other words we are investing approximately £42 000 to prevent one transmission of HIV. Although perhaps economically naive, it raises the question of how much society should be prepared to invest to prevent the thousands of transmissions occurring every year through sexual and needle-sharing transmission.

11. Public health education campaigns

In the autumn of 1986 a major public health education campaign commenced in the UK through posters, a national leaflet drop, and television advertising, with a budget of £20 million ($29 million). The goal of this campaign is to achieve behaviour change and subsequent reduction of the rate of virus transmission. Such strategies are more likely to be successful at a time when the virus is at a very low prevalence within a given community, since the risk of acquiring infection increases as prevalence in the community increases. This is presumably the rationale behind the current campaign in the UK which is directed as much towards heterosexuals as towards high risk groups at a time when the prevalence amongst heterosexuals appears to be very low.[20]

Public health education campaigns may mobilize both inappropriate and appropriate anxiety in the population. For this reason, such campaigns may create considerable demand for individual advice to which resources may need to be committed if intervention is to be effective.

In both the USA and the UK health education has relied considerably on the ingenuity and resources of the voluntary sector. Two-thirds of the total hours worked in the San Francisco AIDS Foundation, the main health education resource in San Francisco, is provided by volunteer labour and 29 per cent of its expenditure is provided from voluntary contributions.[8] In the UK, the Terrence Higgins Trust relies for two-thirds of its income on voluntary donations, and has provided a major national source of individual telephone advice as a back-up to the government health education campaign.

12. Evaluation

It is essential that both public and individual health education strategies are adequately evaluated if their effectiveness in reducing the rate of viral transmission is to be assessed. It is presumably possible for campaigns to achieve behaviour change without reducing the incidence of new infection. Transmission rates will be affected by heterogeneity of sexual behaviour in the population, and rates of viral transmission may slow because of behaviour patterns existing prior to intervention, independent of subsequent changes. The effectiveness of public health campaigns can only be assessed by population-based measures of behaviour change and of rates of virus transmission. Such data, coupled with estimates of infectivity, may help mathematical modellers to chart the future course of the epidemic with greater confidence.

The economist will not only require better epidemic predictions, but must also gather more extensive data on costs of care and relative costs of different care strategies. Any forecasts of future health care use will be limited by the uncertainties surrounding both predictions and calculations of costs.

Finally, the health planner requires both predictions and economic estimates to arrive at policy decisions for care and prevention. The future of the AIDS epidemic depends partly on the existing level of infection and crucially on the future case reproduction rate for HIV infection. Only by measuring that rate, and the ability of health education strategies to affect it, can the best use of limited resources for health care and promotion be made.

References

1 Hardy, A.M., Rauch, K., Echenberg, D., Morgan, W.M., and Curran, J.W. (1986). The economic impact of the first 10 000 cases of Acquired

Immunodeficiency Syndrome in the United States. *Journal of the American Medical Association* **255**, 209–11.

2   Scitovsky, A.A., Cline, M., and Lee, P.R. (1986). Medical care costs of patients with AIDS in San Francisco. *Journal of the American Medical Association* **256**, 3103–6.

3   Seage, G.R., Landers, S., Barry, A., Groopman J., Lamb, G.A., and Epstein, A.M. (1986). Medical care costs of AIDS in Massachusetts. *Journal of the American Medical Association* **256**, 3107–9.

4   Johnson, A.M., Adler, M.W., and Crown, J.M. (1986). The Acquired Immune Deficiency Syndrome and epidemic of infection with Human Immunodeficiency Virus: costs of care and prevention in an inner London District. *British Medical Journal* **293**, 489–92.

5   Marasca, G. and McEvoy, M. (1986). Length of survival of patients with Acquired Immune Deficiency Syndrome in the United States. *British Medical Journal* **292**, 1727–9.

6   Institute of Medicine, National Academy of Sciences (1986). *Costs of health care for HIV related conditions. In: Confronting AIDS: Directions for public health, health care and research*, pp. 155–73. National Academy Press, Washington, DC.

7   Wachter, R.M., Luce, J.M., Turner, J., Volberding, P., and Hopewell P.C. (1986). Intensive care of patients with the Acquired Immunodeficiency Syndrome. Outcome and changing patterns of utilization. *American Review of Respiratory Diseases* **134**, 891–6.

8   Arno, P.S. (1986). The nonprofit sector's response to the AIDS epidemic: community based services in San Francisco. *American Journal of Public Health* **76**, 1325–30.

9   Tillett, H.E. and McEvoy, M. (1986). Reassessment of predicted numbers of AIDS cases in the UK. *Lancet* **ii**, 1104.

10   Green, J., Singer, M., and Winterfield, N. *The AIDS epidemic: a projection of its impact on hospitals 1986–1991. Background paper.* Committee on National Strategy for AIDS, Washington, DC.

11   Jaffe, H.W., Darrow, W.M., Echenberg, D.F., O'Malley, P.M., Getchell, I.P., Kalyanaraman, V.S., Byers, R.H., Drennan, D.P., Braff, E.H., Curran, J.W., and Francis, D.P. (1985). The Acquired Immunodeficiency Syndrome in a cohort of homosexual men. *Annals of Internal Medicine* **103**, 210–4.

12   Who Pays for AIDS? *Nature, London* **321**, 548 (1986).

13   Anderson, F. (1987). Cuts quandary for regions over AIDS funding. *Health Service Journal* **175** (12 Feb 1987).

14   Wells, N. (1986). *The AIDS virus: forecasting its impact.* Office of Health Economics, London.

15   Kristal, A.R. (1986). The impact of the Acquired Immunodeficiency Syndrome on patterns of premature death in New York City. *Journal of the American Medical Association* **255**, 2306–10.

16   Centers for Disease Control (1985). Changes in premature mortality—New York City. *Morbidity and Mortality Weekly Report* **34**, 669–71.

17   Centers for Disease Control (1986). HTLV-III/LAV antibody testing at alternative sites. *Morbidity and Mortality Weekly Report* **35**, 284–7.

18 College of Health (1986). *AIDS and the government*. College of Health, London.
19 Advisory Committee on Dangerous Pathogens (1986). *LAV/HTLV-III—the causative agent of AIDS and related conditions. Revised guidelines*. ACDP Medical Journal, London.
20 Contreras, M. (1987). Who may give blood? *British Journal of Medicine* **294**, 176.

Author index

161

Subject index